COLITIS DIET COOKBOOK

The Complete Guide to Achieving Total Relief from Ulcerative Colitis, Irritable Bowel Syndrome, Crohn's Disease and Other Related Illnesses

Audrey McAllister, MD

Copyright © 2024 Audrey McAllister, MD

this work, individuals agree to comply with the terms and conditions set forth by the publisher regarding copyright protection and usage rights.

Table of Contents

FOREWORD

Colitis can seem like a mysterious and alarming condition, akin to a fever or swelling within the body. Essentially, it involves inflammation of the colon, causing it to swell much like the skin or throat might when irritated or injured. While colitis often stems from an infection and typically subsides once the illness passes, it's crucial to remain vigilant, particularly if gut issues persist for several days, as there could be underlying concerns warranting medical attention.

This inflammation of the large intestine, or colon, manifests as abdominal discomfort, diarrhea, an urgent need to defecate, frequent bowel movements, and sometimes even watery diarrhea, fever, or bloody stools. Colitis is multifaceted in its origins and can be either temporary or persistent, typical of most inflammatory conditions. Treatment strategies aim to address the root cause, with medications potentially reducing swelling and diarrhea in certain types of colitis.

Infections, particularly bacterial ones, represent the most common culprits behind colitis. Various pathogens such as Campylobacter, Salmonella, Shigella, Escherichia coli, and tuberculosis are frequent instigators of gut infections leading to colitis. Among these, Clostridium difficile stands out, causing a severe and sometimes life-threatening form known as pseudomembranous colitis. Additionally, viruses like cytomegalovirus or parasites such as amoebas can also trigger infectious colitis, with amoebic dysentery proving particularly deadly in impoverished regions.

Moreover, individuals with HIV/AIDS are at heightened risk due to opportunistic infections or side effects of antiretroviral therapy. Symptoms of infectious colitis typically include watery, occasionally bloody diarrhea, stomach discomfort, and vomiting, with or without fever accompanying the infection. However, infectious colitis is typically transient, resolving once the underlying infection clears up.

SECTION 1: GETTING TO KNOW COLITIS

olitis, an ailment characterized by inflammation of the colon, presents various challenges to those affected. The colon, responsible for processing digested food into stool, undergoes inflammation, leading to symptoms such as urgent and uncomfortable bowel movements, diarrhea, and sometimes even bloody stools. It's important to note that colitis can manifest differently among individuals, ranging from transient occurrences resulting from infections to chronic forms that persist over time.

The root causes of colitis are diverse, with two primary culprits being ulcerative colitis and Crohn's disease, both categorized under inflammatory bowel diseases (IBD). In these conditions, the lining of the colon becomes inflamed, often triggered by innocuous bacteria and chemicals present in food.

Managing colitis poses a significant challenge, as it often persists as a chronic condition without a definitive cure. However, various medical interventions aim to control and alleviate symptoms, offering relief and improving quality of life for those affected. It's worth noting that colitis typically manifests during specific age ranges, commonly occurring between the ages of 15 and 35, as well as between 55 and 70, highlighting the need for targeted interventions and support across different life stages.

Understanding the Signs and Symptoms of Colitis

• Colitis symptoms vary greatly depending on the underlying causes and may manifest as:

- Abdominal discomfort

- Cramps

- Diarrhea, often accompanied by blood in the stool (a hallmark symptom of colitis).

Associated symptoms can also vary according to the specific cause of colitis and may include:

- Fever

- Chills

- Fatigue

- Dehydration

- Eye inflammation

- Joint swelling

- Canker sores

- Skin inflammation

It's crucial to note that blood in the stool is never a natural occurrence, and seeking medical attention is imperative to determine its cause. Depending on the individual's medical history and physical examination, further diagnostic tests such as blood tests (complete blood count, electrolyte levels, renal function, and inflammatory marker tests), urine and stool samples, colonoscopy, and barium enema may be necessary to pinpoint the etiology of colitis.

Remember, each person's experience with colitis is unique, and a thorough evaluation by healthcare professionals is essential for accurate diagnosis and effective management.

Understanding the Triggers Behind Colitis

The etiology of colitis often remains a mystery, leaving many individuals grappling with uncertainty about the origins of their condition. Colitis can stem from a diverse array of factors, each with its own unique impact on the body and its functioning:

- Infections : Colitis can arise from viral or parasitic infections, which disrupt the delicate balance of the gut microbiome and trigger inflammatory responses.

- Bacterial Food Poisoning : Ingesting contaminated food or water harboring pathogenic bacteria can lead to acute episodes of colitis, characterized by inflammation and damage to the intestinal lining.

- Celiac Disease : For individuals with celiac disease, the ingestion of gluten can trigger an autoimmune response that not only affects the small intestine but can also manifest as colitis.

- Ulcerative Colitis : This chronic inflammatory bowel disease specifically targets the colon and rectum, causing persistent inflammation and ulceration of the intestinal mucosa.

- Ischemic Colitis : Reduced blood flow to the colon, often due to underlying vascular conditions or acute events like thrombosis, can result in ischemic colitis, characterized by tissue damage and inflammation.

- Radiation Exposure : Past radiation therapy directed at the abdomen or pelvis can lead to radiation-induced colitis, a delayed side effect characterized by chronic inflammation and the development of strictures within the large bowel.

- Neonatal Necrotizing Enterocolitis : Premature infants are particularly vulnerable to this serious gastrointestinal condition, which involves inflammation and necrosis of the intestinal tissue.

- Clostridium difficile Infection : This bacterial infection, commonly acquired in healthcare settings, can result in pseudomembranous colitis, now referred to as Clostridioides difficile-associated colitis, characterized by severe inflammation and the formation of pseudomembranes in the colon lining.

These diverse pathways to colitis underscore the complexity of the condition and highlight the importance of tailored treatment approaches that address the underlying causes and individual needs of patients.

SECTION 2: THE DIVERSE FORMS OF COLITIS AND WHAT TRIGGERS THEM

Diving into the realm of colitis reveals a spectrum of variations, each with its own unique triggers and complexities, shaping the landscape of gastrointestinal health in diverse ways. From transient bouts to persistent challenges, the range of colitis encompasses conditions that demand attention, understanding, and tailored care.

At the forefront is infectious colitis, often provoked by viral, parasitic, or bacterial invaders like Salmonella and E. coli, frequently transmitted through contaminated food and water. While typically fleeting, severe cases may necessitate antibiotic intervention to quell the infection's grip.

In a curious twist, pseudomembranous colitis emerges as a subtype of ulcerative colitis, precipitated by the bacterium C. difficile, ironically often induced by antibiotic therapy. This bacterial disruption can upset the delicate microbial balance, paving the way for C. difficile overgrowth and ensuing complications.

Meanwhile, allergic colitis unveils a distinct narrative, notably afflicting breastfeeding infants through maternal transmission of allergenic proteins, predominantly stemming from dairy or soy intolerance. The intricate interplay between maternal diet and infant sensitivities underscores the intricate dynamics of this variant.

Ischemic colitis, a consequence of inadequate blood flow to the intestines, underscores the vascular intricacies underlying gastrointestinal health, often triggered by arterial blockages such as clots, aneurysms, or atherosclerosis.

Inflammatory bowel diseases (IBD) encompass a cluster of conditions, including ulcerative colitis, microscopic colitis, and Crohn's disease, characterized by relentless inflammation within the colon. While their etiology remains elusive, a complex interplay of genetic predisposition and environmental factors paints a multifaceted picture of autoimmune dysfunction.

Radiation colitis serves as a sobering reminder of the collateral damage wrought by cancer treatments, manifesting as a potential aftermath of radiation therapy. While typically transient, its lingering effects underscore the importance of comprehensive supportive care.

Divergent from the others, diversion colitis surfaces as a complication post-colostomy, affecting the dormant segment of the colon. Deprived of its normal function, this overlooked region may suffer malnutrition, posing challenges for a select few navigating this unique terrain.

In the intricate tapestry of colitis, each variant weaves a distinct narrative of challenges and resilience, urging a nuanced approach to management and care, underscoring the imperative of personalized strategies in navigating the complexities of gastrointestinal health.

Exploring the Human Side: Understanding the Health Risks of Colitis

Complications often arise as a result of severe, prolonged chronic colitis. These complications can significantly impact one's health and well-being. Here are some of the potential complications individuals may face:

1. Perforation: Chronic inflammation weakens the walls of the colon, making them more prone to rupture. A colon ulcer can lead to a perforation, creating a hole that allows bacteria from the colon to enter the abdominal cavity, causing peritonitis. In severe cases, bacteria may even enter the bloodstream, leading to septicemia, a life-threatening condition.

2. Toxic Megacolon: Severe inflammation can cause the walls of the colon to dilate, disrupting its normal

muscular movements. This can result in a condition known as toxic megacolon, where food and gas become trapped in the gut, leading to a large bowel obstruction. This obstruction causes painful abdominal distension and increases the risk of rupture.

3. Increased Risk of Colon Cancer: Long-term inflammation is associated with cellular changes in the colon wall, which can occasionally progress to malignant abnormalities. After the first decade of chronic colitis, the risk of colon cancer significantly increases.

It's crucial for individuals with chronic colitis to be aware of these potential complications and to work closely with their healthcare providers to manage their condition effectively. By monitoring symptoms, following treatment plans, and making lifestyle adjustments, individuals can reduce their risk of experiencing these complications and improve their overall quality of life.

Facing the Threat of More Inflammatory Conditions

The heightened risk of developing additional inflammatory illnesses is a significant concern for individuals grappling with inflammatory bowel disease (IBD). Beyond the challenges posed by IBD itself, patients often find themselves navigating a complex landscape of associated health issues. Research has illuminated the interconnected nature of inflammatory disorders, shedding light on how inflammation in one part of the body can influence and exacerbate inflammatory processes elsewhere.

For those with IBD, this heightened susceptibility to other inflammatory conditions underscores the importance of comprehensive health management. Conditions such as osteoarthritis, characterized by joint inflammation, and primary sclerosing cholangitis, involving inflammation in the liver and bile ducts, serve as poignant examples of this interconnectedness. The presence of excessive inflammation in one area may serve as a catalyst for triggering similar processes in other parts of the body.

Understanding this intricate web of interconnected health concerns emphasizes the need for a holistic approach to wellness. Proactive measures to address inflammation and promote overall health become paramount in mitigating the risk of developing additional inflammatory illnesses. By adopting lifestyle strategies, dietary interventions, and targeted medical treatments, individuals can strive to optimize their health outcomes and minimize the impact of inflammatory conditions on their well-being.

SECTION 3: GETTING TO THE BOTTOM OF COLITIS: DIAGNOSIS AND DISCOVERY

Your doctor will kick off the process by chatting with you about your symptoms, digging into when they first showed up, and what your diet and hydration habits were like at that time. They'll also want to know about any medications you're currently taking and any past medical issues you've dealt with. After that, they'll give you a once-over physically before diving into medical tests.

These tests typically include blood work, stool samples, and imaging studies to take a closer look at your colon. Blood tests involve taking a small sample of your blood with a needle and sending it off to a lab for analysis. Stool tests require, well, collecting a stool sample and sending it to a laboratory. The presence of certain proteins in your blood and stool can indicate inflammation and, in some cases, a specific type of infection. Imaging tests can confirm inflammation and provide more detailed insights into your condition.

Endoscopic tests, which involve using a lighted scope to examine the interior of your colon, can be incredibly helpful in determining the type of colitis you're dealing with. Procedures like colonoscopy and flexible sigmoidoscopy allow doctors to gather tissue samples from the inside of your colon through biopsy. Analyzing these tissue samples in the lab can offer crucial information to healthcare providers, helping them tailor your treatment plan to your specific needs.

Colitis Treatments

Addressing Colitis: A Multifaceted Approach

When it comes to treating colitis, the path forward depends greatly on the type and underlying cause of the condition. Fortunately, there are various avenues to explore in the quest for relief and management.

Medications: Your doctor may prescribe a range of medications tailored to your specific situation. This could include antibiotics to combat infections, corticosteroids to tackle inflammation, immunological modifiers to regulate your autoimmune response, and aminosalicylates to address inflammatory bowel disease (IBD).

Dietary Adjustments: Diet plays a crucial role in managing colitis. For those dealing with transient, acute colitis, adopting a low-fiber, easily digestible diet may offer relief. However, for individuals with chronic colitis, a more personalized food plan might be necessary. This could involve avoiding trigger foods known to exacerbate colitis flare-ups while incorporating nutritious alternatives and possibly supplements to ensure adequate nutrition.

Surgical Intervention: In certain cases, particularly with severe forms of colitis like necrotizing enterocolitis, ischemic colitis, and IBD, surgical intervention may be unavoidable. Surgery might be needed to address complications such as bleeding, perforations, or obstructions that cannot be managed through other means.

Navigating colitis involves a comprehensive approach that takes into account medical treatment, dietary considerations, and potentially surgical interventions. By working closely with healthcare professionals and making informed choices, individuals with colitis can strive for better management and improved quality of life.

Can Colitis Be Cured?

Acute colitis, whether triggered by a passing illness, dietary intolerance, or exposure to radiation, typically resolves independently. Infections typically run their course within about a week, while radiation-induced colitis may persist for several months. Some infections, particularly parasite infections, may necessitate antibiotic treatment for resolution.

When it comes to allergic colitis, the condition alleviates once the allergen causing the reaction is removed from the body.

Colitis, as a reaction to a chronic illness, demands therapy for resolution. Ischemic colitis stemming from intestinal ischemic syndrome will persist until blood supply to the colon is restored. Similarly, diversion colitis in individuals with colostomies won't disappear until the colostomy is reversed and the colon functions fully again (through anastomosis surgery). However, these solutions may not be accessible to all individuals.

Chronic colitis resulting from inflammatory bowel disease (IBD) is a lifelong condition that doesn't vanish permanently but can be temporarily alleviated, known as remission. Treatment for IBD focuses on mitigating symptoms and prolonging remission for as long as possible. This remains true even if your colitis stems from another incurable illness. In certain circumstances, surgery may provide a cure.

SECTION 4: WHEN TO REACH OUT TO A PHYSICIAN

If you find yourself grappling with any of the symptoms mentioned below, it's crucial to take them seriously and consider seeking medical assistance:

- Persistent abdominal pain that lingers despite attempts to alleviate it can be indicative of underlying health concerns that warrant attention.

- The presence of blood in your stools or noticing black stools can signal various gastrointestinal issues, ranging from minor to potentially serious conditions. It's essential to have these symptoms evaluated promptly.

- Diarrhea or vomiting that persists beyond what is typical for you may indicate an underlying infection, inflammation, or other digestive disorders that require medical intervention.

- Abdominal swelling or bloating that appears unusual or disproportionate to your typical experiences could signify underlying digestive issues or even more systemic health conditions that need investigation.

Remember, your body communicates with you through symptoms, and ignoring or dismissing them can lead to worsening conditions or complications. Don't hesitate to reach out to your healthcare provider for a thorough evaluation and personalized guidance. Your well-being is paramount, and addressing these symptoms promptly can lead to better management and improved quality of life.

Your Doctor's Evaluation: A Personal Approach to Exams and Assessments

When you step into the healthcare provider's office, expect a comprehensive approach to understanding your health concerns. The journey starts with a thorough physical examination, where the healthcare professional carefully evaluates various aspects of your well-being. This examination is not just about observing external signs; it's about engaging in a dialogue with you to uncover the nuances of your symptoms and experiences.

During this evaluation, you'll find yourself engaged in a conversation that dives deep into your symptoms. These questions are not mere formalities; they're vital pieces of the puzzle that help paint a complete picture of your health. Your healthcare provider will likely inquire about:

1. Duration: How long have you been grappling with these symptoms? The length of time can provide crucial clues about the nature and progression of your condition.

2. Severity: On a scale of one to ten, how would you rate the intensity of your pain or discomfort? This subjective assessment helps gauge the impact of your symptoms on your daily life.

3. Frequency and Duration: How often do you experience discomfort, and how long does it persist? Understanding the frequency and duration of your symptoms can reveal patterns and potential triggers.

4. Gastrointestinal Health: How frequently do you experience diarrhea? This question delves into the specifics of your digestive health, shedding light on potential gastrointestinal issues.

5. Travel and Exposures: Have you recently traveled? Your travel history can offer insights into possible infections or exposures that may contribute to your symptoms.

6. Medication History: Have you taken antibiotics recently? Antibiotic use can disrupt the balance of gut bacteria, potentially leading to gastrointestinal disturbances.

By sharing detailed information about your symptoms and experiences, you empower your healthcare provider to make informed decisions about your care.

Each piece of information you provide serves as a valuable clue in the diagnostic puzzle, guiding the development of a tailored treatment plan that addresses your unique needs. Remember, your voice matters in this process, so don't hesitate to express any concerns or questions you may have—it's all part of working together towards optimal health and well-being.

Finding the Right Diet for Colitis: What Works Best?

Exploring Dietary Paths for Colitis Management

When it comes to managing colitis, the dietary landscape can vary depending on the type of colitis you have and your overall health status. Your doctor, acting as your guide through this journey, may suggest one or more dietary approaches tailored to your specific needs.

1. Low Residue Diet:

In times of acute symptoms or severe flare-ups, a low-residue diet may be recommended. This diet focuses on easy-to-digest foods, limiting fiber and fat intake while prioritizing soft, well-cooked meals. It's particularly beneficial for individuals experiencing transient illness or radiation colitis, providing relief during challenging times.

2. Anti-inflammatory Diet:

Chronic inflammation is a common concern for those with colitis. To address this, your doctor might advise adopting an anti-inflammatory diet, which involves steering clear of highly inflammatory foods, especially those high in sugar and fat. Instead, the emphasis is on incorporating anti-inflammatory options like olive oil, avocados, almonds, and fatty fish such as salmon. The Mediterranean diet, renowned for its anti-inflammatory properties, naturally aligns with this approach.

3. Elimination Diet:

For individuals with inflammatory bowel disease, an elimination diet may be prescribed to identify specific trigger foods aggravating symptoms. This method entails temporarily eliminating certain foods from your diet and gradually reintroducing them to gauge their impact on your digestive system. By pinpointing problematic foods, you can develop a customized, long-term maintenance diet that minimizes discomfort and optimizes gut health.

In essence, navigating the dietary aspects of colitis management involves collaboration between you and your healthcare team. Through careful consideration and experimentation with different dietary strategies, you can uncover the approaches that best support your health and well-being on your journey towards managing colitis effectively.

SECTION 5: NOURISHING MEALS FOR COLITIS

ANTI-COLITIS BREAKFAST RECIPES

Chocolate Strawberry Crepes

Things You Need

for 2 servings

2 cups all-purpose flour (250 g)

3 eggs

¼ cup butter (55 g), melted

3 tablespoons granulated sugar

3 cups milk (720 mL)

½ cup hazelnut spread (115 g)

10 strawberries, sliced

powdered sugar, to Garnish

Instructions

In a large bowl, combine flour, eggs, butter, and sugar, stirring until ingredients are slightly mixed.

Add the milk ½ cup (120 ml) at a time, stirring vigorously, making sure the milk is completely incorporated into the batter and that the batter is smooth before adding more milk.

Repeat with the rest of the milk. The batter should be very liq uidy and have no lumps.

In a pan over medium heat, pour ⅓ cup (95 grams) of the batter in the center and swirl the batter around the edges of the pan until set.

To know when the crepe is ready to flip, lift up one of the edges about ⅓ of the way. The bottom side should be golden brown. Flip the crepe.

Cook until the edges are starting to slightly crisp.

Remove from heat and cover with a paper towel to make sure the crepes stay moist.

Spread half of the chocolate hazelnut spread on half of the crepe.

Lay half of the strawberries on the chocolate spread.

Fold the other half of the crepe on top of the strawberries, then fold the crepe in half.

Repeat with the other crepe.

Enjoy!

Blueberry Overnight Oats

 Things You Need

for 2 servings

⅔ cup rolled oats (65 g)

⅔ cup milk (160 mL), of your choice

½ cup vanilla greek yogurt (120 g)

½ teaspoon vanilla extract

1 teaspoon chia seed, optional

½ teaspoon cinnamon

2 teaspoons honey

blueberry

⅓ cup graham cracker (30 g), crushed

Instructions

In a mason jar or sealable container, add the oats, milk, yogurt, vanilla extract, chia seeds, cinnamon, blueberries, and graham crackers, and stir together.

Seal and place in the refrigerator overnight for up to five days.

Top with additional blueberries, if desired.

Enjoy!

Banana Muffin Mug

Things You Need

for 1 muffin

1 banana

¼ cup oat flour (20 g)

½ teaspoon baking powder

2 tablespoons honey

1 egg white

½ teaspoon cinnamon

Instructions

Mix together egg white and honey in a greased coffee mug.

Add oat flour, baking powder, and cinnamon, and mix until combined.

Add in fresh bananas.

Microwave on high for 90 seconds (times may vary).

Enjoy!

Mixed Berry French Toast

Things You Need

for 2 servings

4 slices bread

Egg Wash

4 eggs

1 cup milk (240 mL)

1 tablespoon vanilla

1 tablespoon cinnamon

Mixed Berry Sauce

2 cups mixed berries (200 g), blueberries, raspberries, and blackberries

2 tablespoons lemon juce

⅓ cup granulated sugar (65 g)

Garnish

confectioners sugar, optional

Instructions

Whisk eggs, cinnamon, vanilla and milk together in medium-large bowl to create egg wash.

Dunk bread in egg wash.

Melt butter in a skillet on medium-low heat and cook bread for 2-3 minutes.

Mix berries, sugar, and lemon juice in medium pan over low heat crushing and stirring berries until they form a thick sauce.

Lay out slices and spread compote in between each slice then on top. Garnish with confectioners sugar (optional).

Enjoy!

Dark Chocolate Peanut Butter Banana Protein Smoothie

Things You Need

for 2 servings

1 ½ cups water (360 mL), or yogurt or milk of choice

¼ cup peanut butter (60 g)

1 scoop chocolate protein powder

1 tablespoon dark chocolate cocoa powder

2 bananas, frozen

Instructions

Put all ingredients into a blender and mix until smooth.

Enjoy!

Steak And Eggs Hash

Things You Need

for 4 servings

2 lb yukon gold potato (910 g), peeled and cut into 1/2 in (1 1/2 cm)

cold water, for cooking potatoes

1 ½ tablespoons kosher salt, divided

1 top sirloin steak

1 ½ teaspoons freshly ground black pepper, divided

2 tablespoons unsalted butter, divided

1 tablespoon canola oil

½ small yellow onion, thinly sliced

8 oz cremini mushroom (225 g), steemed and q uartered

1 small red bell pepper, seeded and diced

1 teaspoon fresh oregano, chopped

1 cup cherry tomato (200 g), halved

4 large eggs

1 tablespoon fresh parsley, minced \

Instructions

Add the potatoes to a large pot and fill with enough cold water to cover by 1 inch (2 ½ cm). Season with 1½ teaspoons of salt and bring to a boil over medium-high heat. Boil for 5 minutes, then drain and run under cold water to stop the potatoes from cooking further. Dry the potatoes with paper towels and set aside.

Place a rack in the lower third of the oven. Preheat the oven to 350°F (180°C)

Blot the steak dry with a paper towel and season on both sides with 1½ teaspoons of salt and 1 teaspoon black pepper.

Heat a 10-inch (25 cm) cast iron skillet over high heat until smoking. Reduce the heat to medium-high. Add 1 tablespoon of butter and the canola oil to the pan and melt the butter completely, about 1 minute. Add the seasoned steak and cook, without disturbing, for 2 minutes on each side. The steak will be rare, but will finish cooking in the oven. Transfer to a cutting board to rest for at least 5 minutes before slicing into ¼-inch (6 mm) strips.

Reduce the heat to medium and melt the remaining tablespoon of butter in the same skillet. Add the onion, mushrooms, red bell pepper, and ½ teaspoon of salt. Cook, stirring occasionally, until the onions are slightly caramelized and the mushrooms have released their liquid, 8–10 minutes.

Add the potatoes to the skillet and season with the remaining teaspoon of salt, ¼ teaspoon black pepper, and the oregano. Stir to combine and cook, without disturbing, for 4 minutes, until the potatoes are golden brown and crisp on one side. Add the cherry tomatoes and stir to combine.

Make 4 wells in the hash using the back of a spoon and carefully crack an egg into each well.

Scatter the sliced steak on top of the hash and transfer to the oven. Bake for 10 minutes, or until the egg whites are set but the yolks are still runny.

Remove the hash from the oven and season with the remaining ¼ teaspoon pepper. Garnish with the parsley.

Serve warm.

Enjoy!

Healthy Dark Chocolate Pancakes

Things You Need

for 4 servings

2 bananas

2 eggs

½ cup q uick-cook oats (70 g)

2 tablespoons dark cocoa powder

¼ cup dark chocolate chips (50 g)

¼ teaspoon salt

Instructions

Mash bananas in a large bowl until smooth. Mix in eggs until well combined, then mix in remaining ingredients.

Heat a skillet to medium and add in a scoop of the pancake batter. Smooth out to form an even layer. Cook for about 2-3 minutes until you start to see bubbles releasing from the top of the batter. Flip and cook until the other side is golden brown, about 1-2 minutes.

Garnish your pancakes with your favorite toppings! We used fresh strawberries and maple syrup.

Enjoy!

Spiced Chorizo And Tomato Shakshuka

Things You Need

for 4 servings

1 tablespoon olive oil

¾ cup chorizo (100 g), chopped into 1/4 in pieces

1 medium onion, chopped

2 cloves garlic, chopped

red bell pepper, chopped into 1/2 in (1 1/4 cm) pieces

1 tablespoon paprika

½ teaspoon ground cumin

¼ teaspoon ground pepper

1 pinch sea salt

5 lb tomato (2.4 g), chopped

4 eggs

½ cup feta cheese (50 g), crumbled

¼ cup fresh parsley (15 g)

Instructions

Heat oil in a frying pan over medium heat.

Add chorizo, onion, garlic, and red bell pepper, cooking for 2–-3 minutes, or until fragrant.

Add paprika, ground cumin, pepper, and salt. Stir to combine, cooking for 6–-8 minutes, or until the vegetables begin to soften.

Pour tinned tomatoes into the skillet, reduce heat, and let simmer for 20–-25 minutes, or until the sauce begins to thicken.

Using the back of a spoon, make 4 wells in the tomato sauce. Crack an egg into each well.

Cover the skillet with a lid, and cook for 6–-8 minutes, or until eggs are cooked.

Top with crumbled feta and chopped parsley.

Enjoy!

Almond Butter Honey Oat Bars

Things You Need

for 8 servings

2 cups rolled oats (160 g)

⅔ cup almond butter (160 g), or nut butter of choice

¼ cup honey (85 g), or maple syrup

Instructions

In a medium bowl, add oats, nut butter, and honey or maple syrup, and mix until well combined.

Spray baking dish with cooking spray. Pour in mixture and spread evenly.

Cover and place in freezer until firm.

Cut into bars. Keep in the fridge until ready to eat.

Enjoy!

Spicy Fried Egg Avocado Toast

Things You Need

for 1 serving

bread, toasted

½ avocado, mashed

salt, to taste

pepper, to taste

1 egg, fried to preference

½ teaspoon Sriracha

Instructions

Mash half of an avocado. Add salt and pepper, to taste. Mix until well combined.

Spread the mashed avocado evenly across toast.

Top with the fried egg, and drizzle with Sriracha.

Enjoy!

Strawberry Shortcake Sheet Pan Pancakes

Things You Need

for 4 servings

4 cups pancake mix (480 g)

4 eggs

2 cups milk (480 mL)

6 oz cream cheese (170 g), cubed

1 cup strawberry (150 g), sliced

Instructions

Preheat oven to 425°F (220°C).

Pour pancake mix, milk, and eggs into a bowl and mix just until combined.

Pour batter onto a parchment paper-lined baking sheet and spread to the edges.

Place cream cheese on top of the batter, followed by the strawberry slices.

Bake for 15 minutes, or until golden brown.

Cut into squares and serve immediately, or freeze up to 1 month. To reheat, place on a microwave-safe plate and heat for 20 seconds per pancake on the plate.

Enjoy!

Tater Tot Breakfast Pizza

Things You Need

for 4 servings

4 cups tater tot (345 g)

7 eggs

½ cup bacon bits (110 g)

½ avocado

½ cup shredded cheddar cheese (50 g)

½ cup shredded mozzarella cheese (50 g)

butter

pepper, to taste

Instructions

Pour the tater tots in a large mixing bowl. Microwave for one minute and forty-five seconds (or until soft)

Add one egg to the softened tater tots and mix.

Grease a cast-iron pan with butter, then pour the tater-tot mixture into the pan and spread it out to create a crust.

Bake the crust for 15 minutes at 400°F (200°C).

Remove from the oven, then add ½ of the cheddar cheese, ½ of the mozzarella cheese, and ½ of the bacon bits to the base of the crust.

Crack the rest of the eggs evenly over the top of the crust, then top with the rest of the cheese and bacon bits.

Bake for 15 more minutes at 400°F (200°C).

Top with avocado slices and pepper.

Enjoy!

Sweet Potato Breakfast Boats

Things You Need

for 4 servings

2 large sweet potatoes

4 large eggs

salt, to taste

black pepper, to taste

Assorted Fillings And Toppings

spinach

tomato, diced

1 head broccoli floret

shredded cheddar cheese

white onion, diced

red bell pepper, diced

bacon, cooked and crumbled

sriracha sauce

avocado

Instructions

Use a fork to pierce holes all over the sweet potatoes.

Preheat oven to 400°F (200°C).

Microwave the potatoes for 7 minutes until they have softened significantly.

Slice the potatoes in half and use a spoon to scrape out the inner flesh, making sure to leave at least a ¼-inch (6 mm) thick border on each side, saving the scooped out potato parts to use for side dishes.

Transfer the potatoes to a parchment paper-lined baking sheet.

Fill each of the potatoes with 1 egg and an assortment of fillings for whatever flavor combinations you'd like. Season each potatoes with salt and pepper.

Bake for 8-12 minutes, until the egg has cooked to preferred doneness.

Top the potatoes and side dishes with your choice of topping and garnishes and serve.

Enjoy!

Banana Chocolate Chip Pancakes

Things You Need

for 4 servings

4 cups pancake mix (480 g)

4 eggs

2 cups milk (480 mL)

1 banana, sliced

¾ cup chocolate chips (130 g)

Instructions

Preheat oven to 425°F (220°C).

Pour pancake mix, milk, and eggs into a bowl and mix just until combined.

Pour batter onto a parchment-lined baking sheet and spread to the edges.

Place banana slices on top of the batter, followed by the chocolate chips.

Bake for 15 minutes, or until golden brown.

Cut into sq uares and serve immediately, or freeze up to 1 month. To reheat, place on a microwave-safe plate and heat for 20 seconds per pancake on the plate.

Enjoy!

Mixed Berry Sheet Pan Pancakes

Things You Need

for 4 servings

4 cups pancake mix (480 g)

4 eggs

2 cups milk (480 mL)

1 cup strawberry (150 g), sliced

½ cup blueberry (50 g)

1 cup raspberry (125 g)

Instructions

Preheat oven to 425°F (220°C).

Pour pancake mix, milk, and eggs into a bowl and mix just until combined.

Pour batter onto a parchment-lined baking sheet and spread to the edges.

Place strawberry slices on top of the batter, followed by the blueberries and raspberries.

Bake for 15 minutes, or until golden brown.

Cut into sq uares and serve immediately, or freeze up to 1 month.

To reheat, place on a microwave-safe plate and heat for 20 seconds per pancake on the plate.

Enjoy!

Protein-Packed Breakfast Bars

Things You Need

for 24 bars

Base

¼ cup flax meal (40 g)

¾ cup water (180 mL)

6 cups rolled oats (540 g)

6 cups q uinoa (1 kg), cooked

4 teaspoons baking powder

1 teaspoon salt

1 cup maple syrup (220 g)

½ cup refined coconut oil (120 mL), melted

2 teaspoons vanilla extract

4 ripe bananas, mashed

Fillings

Peanut Butter Chocolate Chip

6 tablespoons peanut butter

5 tablespoons mini chocolate chips

Apple Cinnamon

¾ cup gala apple (90 g), diced

6 tablespoons walnuts, chopped

1 ½ tablespoons cinnamon

¼ teaspoon nutmeg

Carrot Cake

¾ cup carrot (30 g), grated

3 teaspoons cinnamon

¼ teaspoon nutmeg

3 tablespoons almond butter

Mixed Berry

3 tablespoons almond butter

⅓ cup Strawberries (55 g), diced

⅓ cup raspberries (40 g)

⅓ cup blueberries (40 g)

nonstick cooking spray

Instructions

Preheat the oven to 375°F (190°C).

To make the flax eggs, combine the flax meal and water in a small bowl and mix well. Set aside for 10 minutes to gel.

In a large bowl, combine the oats, q uinoa, baking powder, salt, maple syrup, coconut oil, vanilla, flax eggs, and bananas, and mix until well-combined.

Divide the base dough equally between 4 medium bowls.

Add the peanut butter and chocolate chips to 1 bowl and mix until combined.

Add the apple, walnuts, cinnamon, and nutmeg to another bowl and mix until combined.

Add the carrots, cinnamon, nutmeg, and almond butter to another bowl and mix until combined.

Add the almond butter, strawberries, raspberries, and blueberries to the last bowl and mix until combined.

Grease 2 9x13-inch (23x33-cm) baking pans with nonstick spray. Transfer the bar mixtures to the pans, packing each mixture into half of a pan with a spoon or spatula.

Bake for 25-30 minutes, until the edges are slightly golden brown.

Remove the pans from the oven and let the bars cool for 20 minutes, then refrigerate for at least 30 minutes, or up to 5 days. Gently cut each flavor into 6 bars, then remove from the pans with a spatula.

Enjoy!

Simple Shakshuka

Things You Need

for 4 servings

olive oil, drizzle

1 cup yellow onion (150 g), diced

1 orange bell pepper, diced

salt, to taste

pepper, to taste

½ teaspoon cumin

½ teaspoon paprika

3 cloves garlic, chopped

28 oz crushed tomatoes (795 g), 1 can

1 bay leaf

1 ½ cups fresh baby kale (100 g)

4 large eggs

¼ cup feta cheese (25 g), crumble

bread, toasted, for serving

Instructions

Heat a large cast iron skillet over medium-low heat.

Once the pan is hot, add the olive oil and swirl to coat the pan. Add the onion, bell pepper, salt, and pepper. Sauté 5 minutes, or until the onion is almost translucent.

Add the cumin, paprika, and garlic. Sauté 2-3 minutes, or until the garlic is slightly brown.

Pour in the crushed tomatoes and add the bay leaf. Simmer for 10-15 minutes, or until the mixture has thickened.

Stir in the baby kale until wilted.

Reduce the heat to low, then carefully crack the eggs into the sauce. Cover and simmer until the egg whites are set, about 10-12 minutes.

Top with the feta cheese and remove the pan from the heat.

Enjoy!

Breakfast Veggie Pocket

Things You Need

for 1 serving

2 teaspoons olive oil

½ red bell pepper, sliced

¼ cup canned black bean (40 g), drained and rinsed

¼ cup frozen corn (45 g), thawed

½ small yellow onion, thinly sliced

2 eggs

¼ teaspoon salt

¼ teaspoon ground black pepper

¼ cup shredded cheddar cheese (25 g)

1 whole wheat tortilla, medium

Instructions

Heat olive oil in a nonstick skillet over medium heat.

Add the bell pepper, black beans, corn, and onions, and cook until caramelized, about 5 minutes.

Remove the vegetables from the pan and set aside.

Reduce heat to low, and eggs, and sprinkle with salt and pepper. Cook, stirring constantly, until barely set, about 2 minutes.

Place the vegetables, scrambled eggs, and cheese in the center of a tortilla, and fold the sides into the center, completely covering the filling.

Add the q uesadilla, seam side down, to the skillet and cook over medium heat until the outside is toasted and cheese is melted.

Enjoy!

Berry-Stuffed French Toast For Two

Things You Need

for 2 servings

Filling

1 cup raspberry (125 g)

1 cup blackberry (125 g)

2 tablespoons maple syrup, divided

1 tablespoon black raspberry liq ueur

4 oz cream cheese (115 g), softened

French Toast

4 slices brioche bread

½ cup whole milk (120 mL)

1 large egg, beaten

2 tablespoons black raspberry liq ueur

½ teaspoon salt

2 tablespoons butter

Whipped Cream

½ cup heavy cream (120 mL)

1 tablespoon maple syrup

Instructions

Make the filling: Add the raspberries, blackberries, black raspberry liq ueur, and 1 tablespoon of maple syrup to a large bowl. Stir and let sit for 10 minutes for the berries to macerate.

In a medium bowl, mix together the cream cheese and remaining tablespoon of maple syrup until smooth.

Spread the filling evenly over the 4 slices of bread. Arrange some of the berries on 2 slices of the bread and top with the other slices of bread. Press to seal the pieces together.

In a shallow dish, whisk together the milk, egg, black raspberry liq ueur, and salt.

Melt the butter on a griddle or in a large skillet over medium heat. Quickly dip both sides of the bread pockets in the milk mixture, then transfer to the pan and fry on each side for about 3 minutes, until golden brown.

In a large bowl, beat the heavy cream until soft peaks form. Add the maple syrup and continue beating until the cream holds medium peaks.

Serve the stuffed French toast with a dollop of maple whipped cream and a scoop of macerated berries with their soaking liq uid.

Enjoy!

Crispy Cheesy Hash Brown Egg Bake

Things You Need

for 6 servings

4 lb russet potato (1.8 kg)

salt, to taste

pepper, to taste

1 tablespoon garlic powder

¼ teaspoon cayenne pepper

1 teaspoon onion powder

1 cup shredded parmesan cheese (100 g)

¼ cup olive oil (60 mL)

12 slices cheddar cheese, cut into 1x3in (2x7 cm) strips

12 slices deli ham, cut into 1x3in (2x7 cm) strips

6 large eggs

fresh chive, chopped, for garnish

Instructions

Preheat the oven to 400°F (200°C). Grease a 9x13-inch (23x33-cm) baking dish with non-stick cooking spray

Peel the potatoes, then shred on the large holes of a box grater. Transfer to a large bowl of water and swirl around to remove excess starch.

Drain and rinse, then place the potatoes in a clean kitchen towel and squeeze until they're completely dry.

Add the shredded potatoes to a clean, large bowl with the salt, pepper, garlic powder, cayenne, onion powder, Parmesan cheese, and olive oil. Toss until fully combined.

Transfer the potato mixture to the baking dish. Spread evenly.

Bake for 1½ hours, or until the potatoes are tender throughout and golden brown on the top and bottom.

Press the bottom of a glass into the potato mixture to create 6 evenly spaced wells.

Shingle slices of cheddar cheese and ham around the wells, then crack an egg into each one.

Bake for 15 minutes more, or until the cheese melts and the egg whites are set. The egg yolks should still be slightly soft.

Serve and sprinkle with chives, if desired.

Enjoy!

ANTI-COLITIS LUNCH RECIPES

Loaded Baked Potato Soup

Things You Need

for 6 servings

4 lb russet potato (1.8 g), washed

1 tablespoon olive oil

1 teaspoon salt

½ teaspoon pepper

1 onion, diced

3 cloves garlic

3 tablespoons butter

¼ cup flour (30 g)

2 ½ cups chicken broth (590 mL)

8 oz cream cheese (225 g)

Garnish

shredded cheese

bacon, diced

fresh chive, chopped

Instructions

Preheat your oven to 425°F (220°C).

On a parchment paper-lined baking sheet, rub potatoes with salt, pepper, and olive oil.

Bake in preheated oven for 40-50 minutes.

Once cooled, peel and mash potatoes, and set aside.

Heat oil in large pot over a medium-high heat.

Add onion and garlic. Cook until translucent and garlic is fragant, about 5 minutes.

Add butter and melt.

Bring in flour and stir until mixture is lightly browned.

Add in the chicken broth and cream cheese. Stir until fully incorporated

Add in the mashed potatoes and combine.

Season with salt and pepper.

Garnish bowl with shredded cheese, bacon, and chives.

Enjoy!

Cashew Chicken Stir-Fry

Things You Need

for 4 servings

6 tablespoons soy sauce

1 tablespoon hoisin sauce

1 tablespoon rice vinegar

2 tablespoons honey

1 teaspoon sesame oil

½ tablespoon ginger, minced

2 cloves garlic, minced

¾ lb chicken breast (340 g), cut into 1-inch (2 1/2 cm) pieces

salt, to taste

pepper, to taste

1 tablespoon cornstarch

1 tablespoon sesame oil

4 cups broccoli floret (600 g)

1 red bell pepper, cut into 1-inch (2 1/2 cm) pieces

¾ cup raw cashew (95 g)

½ cup water (120 mL)

brown rice, to serve

Instructions

In a medium bowl, combine the soy sauce, hoisin sauce, rice vinegar, honey, sesame oil, ginger, and garlic. Set aside.

In a medium bowl, season the chicken with salt, pepper, and cornstarch.

Heat a 9.5" fry pan over medium-high heat and add sesame oil.

Add the chicken and cook for 5-6 minutes, or until the chicken begins to brown.

Remove chicken and set aside in a separate bowl.

Add the broccoli and bell peppers, and cook for 2-3 minutes.

Add the chicken, cashews and sauce. Stir together and allow sauce to thicken.

Remove from heat and serve over brown rice.

Enjoy!

Chickpea Sweet Potato Stew

Things You Need

for 4 servings

2 tablespoons refined coconut oil

1 small onion, diced

3 cloves garlic, minced

1 teaspoon ginger, minced

1 tablespoon sweet paprika

½ teaspoon cumin

¼ teaspoon dried coriander

⅛ teaspoon cayenne

15 oz chickpeas (425 g), 1 can, drained and rinsed

2 cups sweet potato (400 g), peeled and diced

15 oz fire roasted crushed tomato (425 g), 1 can

3 cups vegetable broth (720 mL)

5 oz fresh spinach (140 g)

Instructions

In large pot or Dutch oven, heat the coconut oil over medium heat. Once the oil begins to shimmer, add the onion and cook for 4-5 minutes, or until the onion is semi-translucent.

Add the garlic and ginger, and cook for 2-3 more minutes, until fragrant. Then add the sweet paprika, cumin, coriander, and cayenne and cook for 2 more minutes, until fragrant.

Add the chickpeas, sweet potatoes, crushed tomatoes, and vegetable broth, and bring to a boil. Reduce the heat to medium-low and simmer for 15-20 minutes, or until the sweet potatoes are tender.

Add the spinach and stir until wilted.

Serve immediately.

Enjoy!

One-Pot Mexican Quinoa

Things You Need

for 4 servings

1 cup quinoa (170 g), rinsed

1 ½ cups water (360 mL), or vegetable broth

1 ¼ cups salsa (325 g)

1 tablespoon cumin

15 oz black beans (425 g), 1 can, drained and rinsed

1 cup frozen corn (175 g), defrosted

salt, to taste

olive oil, to taste

1 avocado, mashed

1 clove garlic, minced

2 teaspoons lemon juice

3 tablespoons olive oil

salt, to taste

pepper, to taste

4 tablespoons water

tortilla, to serve, optional

Instructions

In a medium saucepan, combine q uinoa and water, and bring to a boil over high heat. Reduce heat to low, cover with a lid, and simmer for 10 minutes.

Add in salsa and cumin, and cover for 5 more minutes or until q uinoa is fluffy.

Add in black beans, corn, salt, and olive oil, and stir until combined.

For the avocado dressing, combine avocado, garlic, lemon juice, olive oil, salt, and pepper in liq uid measuring cup and whisk until smooth.

Whisk in water a little bit at a time until desired consistency is reached. 6. For extra smooth consistency, process all ingredients in blender or food processor.

Portion out into 4 containers and refrigerate for up to 5 days.

Enjoy!

One-pan Roasted Chicken And Sweet Potatoes

Things You Need

for 1 serving

1 small sweet potato, diced

1 lemon, sliced, seeds removed

1 cup green beans (360 g), trimmed

1 tablespoon olive oil

1 tablespoon fresh rosemary, chopped

1 tablespoon fresh thyme, chopped

1 clove garlic, minced

½ teaspoon salt, plus more to season

¼ teaspoon ground black pepper, plus more to season

1 boneless, skinless chicken breast

¼ teaspoon paprika

Instructions

Preheat oven to 375°F (190°C).

Add the sweet potatoes, lemon slices, green beans, olive oil, rosemary, thyme, garlic, salt, and pepper to a large bowl (or parchment paper-lined sheet tray) and toss until fully coated.

Season the chicken breast with salt, pepper, and paprika.

Transfer to a parchment paper-lined sheet tray and place the chicken breast on top of the vegetables (if you tossed your vegetables in a bowl).

Bake until vegetables are tender and chicken is cooked through, about 20 minutes.

Enjoy!

Easy Vegan Pasta Salad

Things You Need

for 4 servings

8 oz dried pasta (225 g), cooked

15 oz chickpeas (425 g), 1 can, drained and rinsed

1 cup broccoli floret (150 g), steamed

½ cup carrot (60 g), shredded

½ cup red onion (75 g), sliced

¼ cup fresh parsley (10 g)

¼ cup olive oil (60 mL)

¼ cup red wine vinegar (60 mL)

1 clove garlic, minced

1 teaspoon dried oregano

salt, to taste

pepper, to taste

1 ½ cups cherry tomatoes (300 g)

Instructions

In a large mixing bowl, combine pasta, chickpeas, grape tomatoes, broccoli, carrots, red onion, and parsley.

In a small liq uid measuring cup, combine olive oil, red wine vinegar, garlic, oregano, salt, and pepper, and whisk to combine.

Pour dressing over pasta salad and stir until evenly distributed.

Transfer pasta salad into 4 containers and refrigerate for up to 5 days.

Enjoy!

Chickpea Salad Sandwich

Things You Need

for 3 servings

15 oz chickpeas (425 g), 1 can, drained and rinsed

¼ cup red onion (40 g), diced

½ red bell pepper, diced

3 tablespoons vegan mayonnaise

½ teaspoon dijon mustard

½ teaspoon garlic powder

½ teaspoon onion powder

salt, to taste

pepper, to taste

1 tablespoon fresh dill, chopped

leafy green, to serve

bread, sliced, to serve

Instructions

In a medium mixing bowl, add chickpeas and mash with potato masher until a chunky texture is reached.

Add the red onion, red pepper, vegan mayo, Dijon mustard, garlic powder, onion powder, salt, pepper, and dill, and stir until well combined.

Store chickpea salad in refrigerator for up to five days. To assemble sandwich, spread mixture onto bread and top with leafy greens of choice.

Wrap in parchment paper and secure with rubber band.

Enjoy!

Easy Salmon Dinner

Things You Need

for 2 servings

1 lb potato (455 g)

olive oil, to taste

salt, to taste

pepper, to taste

3 tablespoons lemon juice

2 cloves garlic, minced

½ teaspoon onion powder

½ teaspoon paprika

½ teaspoon dried thyme

½ teaspoon dried parsley

2 tablespoons honey

2 salmon fillets

1 bunch asparagus

6 slices lemon

4 sprigs fresh thyme

Instructions

Preheat oven to 400°F (200°C)

Add potatoes to a parchment paper-lined baking sheet.

Season with olive oil, thyme, salt, and pepper.

Bake for 20 minutes.

To prepare salmon marinade, combine lemon juice, garlic, onion powder, paprika, thyme, parsley, and honey, and stir until evenly combined.

On the same baking tray, push the potatoes to one side of the tray and add salmon and asparagus.

Season the salmon and asparagus with olive oil, salt, and pepper. Brush the marinade on the salmon.

Top salmon with lemon slices and thyme springs.

Bake for 12-14 minutes or until salmon is cooked.

Enjoy!

Honey Mustard Chicken Salad

Things You Need

for 4 servings

⅓ cup honey (115 g)

¼ cup dijon mustard (65 g)

2 tablespoons olive oil

2 cloves garlic, minced

2 teaspoons salt

1 teaspoon pepper

4 boneless, skinless chicken thighs

¼ cup bacon (60 g), chopped

4 cups romaine lettuce (300 g), chopped

1 cup cherry tomatoes (200 g), halved

¼ red onion, sliced

1 avocado, pitted and sliced

Instructions

In a small bowl or liq uid measuring cup, mix the honey, mustard, oil, garlic, salt, and pepper.

Place the chicken thighs in a dish and pour the marinade over the chicken, reserving half for later.

Flip the chicken thighs over, fully covering them in the marinade.

Cover the dish with plastic wrap and refrigerate for 30 minutes to an hour.

Heat a large skillet over medium heat, and place the chicken thighs in the pan.

Cook for five minutes on each side, or until the chicken is cooked through.

Remove the chicken and set aside.

Wipe the pan clean and place back on the heat.

Add the chopped bacon to the pan and cook until crispy, about ten minutes.

Transfer the bacon to a paper towel-lined plate to drain.

Add three tablespoons of water to the reserved marinade and stir to combine.

Slice the chicken into strips.

Add the romaine, cherry tomatoes, red onion, avocado, cooked bacon, and chicken to a bowl and drizzle with the remaining honey mustard dressing.

Enjoy!

Easy Honey-Mustard Chicken Meal Prep

Things You Need

for 4 servings

1 cup sweet potato (200 g), diced

1 cup red potato (225 g), diced

1 cup red onion (150 g), chopped

1 cup brussel sprout (100 g), quartered

1 cup green beans (360 g), chopped

1 cup carrot (120 g), chopped

olive oil, to taste

salt, to taste

pepper, to taste

½ tablespoon dried thyme

1 tablespoon fresh rosemary, chopped

¼ cup dijon mustard (60 g)

¼ cup honey (85 g)

3 cloves garlic, minced

4 chicken thighs

Instructions

Preheat the oven to 400°F (200°C) and line a baking sheet with parchment paper.

Place the sweet potato, red potato, red onion, Brussels sprouts, green beans, and carrots on the baking sheet in separate piles.

Drizzle everything with olive oil, then sprinkle with salt, pepper, thyme, and rosemary. Rub the seasoning into the vegetables until evenly coated and spread flat on the baking sheet, keeping the vegetables separate. Set aside.

In a small bowl, combine the mustard, honey, garlic, salt, and pepper, and whisk until smooth. Set aside.

Place the chicken thighs skin-side down in a greased cast-iron skillet. Season with salt and pepper, then brush generously with the honey-mustard sauce. Flip the chicken thighs over and repeat, seasoning with salt and pepper, then brushing with the rest of the honey-mustard sauce.

Place the vegetables and the chicken in the oven on separate racks. Bake for 30 minutes or until chicken reaches an internal temperature of 165°F (75°C) . (Optional: Remove the vegetables once cooked and broil the chicken for 1-2 minutes, or until the skin crisps up.)

Let everything cool, then distribute into resealable containers, mixing up the combination of vegetables so that you get something a little different each day.

Cover and refrigerate for up to 4 days.

Enjoy!

Orange Cauliflower "Chicken"

Things You Need

for 4 servings

nonstick cooking spray, for greasing

2 cups non dairy milk (480 mL)

2 cups all purpose flour (250 g)

2 teaspoons kosher salt

1 cauliflower, cut into 1 1/2 inch (3 cm) florets

1 tablespoon canola oil

3 cloves garlic, minced

1 piece fresh ginger, minced

¼ teaspoon red pepper flakes

½ cup orange juice (120 mL)

½ cup brown sugar (100 g)

¼ cup distilled white vinegar (60 mL)

¼ cup soy sauce (60 mL)

2 tablespoons cornstarch

2 tablespoons cold water

1 teaspoon sesame oil

white rice, for serving

3 scallions, thinly sliced, for garnish

Instructions

Preheat the oven to 450°F (230°C). Line a baking sheet with parchment paper and grease with nonstick spray.

In a medium bowl, whisk together the non-dairy milk, flour, and salt.

One at a time, dip each cauliflower floret in the batter to coat, letting any excess batter drip off. Arrange the battered cauliflower on the prepared baking sheet, making sure they aren't touching one another. Lightly spray with cooking spray.

Bake for 30–35 minutes, until the coating is crispy and beginning to brown.

While the cauliflower is baking, make the sauce: Heat the canola oil in a medium skillet over medium heat. When the oil is shimmering, add the garlic, ginger, and red pepper flakes. Cook for 2–3 minutes, until fragrant, stirring freq uently to prevent burning.

Add the orange juice, brown sugar, vinegar, and soy sauce. Cook for 2–3 minutes, until the brown sugar is dissolved and the mixture begins to simmer.

In a small bowl, stir together the cornstarch and cold water with a fork.

Add the slurry to the sauce, stirring to combine. Simmer for another 2 minutes, until the sauce thickens. Mix in the sesame oil, then transfer the sauce to a large bowl.

Toss the hot cauliflower florets in the sauce until well coated.

Serve the cauliflower over rice and garnish with the scallions.

Enjoy!

Shrimp & Avocado Tostadas

Things You Need

for 6 tostadas

6 corn tortillas

olive oil, to taste

1 lb shrimp (455 g), peeled and deveined

1 cup english cucumber (135 g), diced

1 cup tomato (200 g), diced

1 avocado, diced

1 cup red onion (150 g), diced

1 lemon, juiced

1 lime, juiced

1 tablespoon fresh cilantro, chopped

salt, to taste

1 serrano pepper, finely chopped, optional

Instructions

Preheat oven to 425°F (220°C).

Lay the corn tortillas on a parchment paper-lined baking sheet and lightly brush both sides with olive oil.

Bake the tortillas for 5 minutes and then flip them over continue baking another 5 minutes. The tostadas should be brown and crispy. Set the pan aside to cool.

Roughly chop the shrimp and transfer to a bowl.

Add the cucumber, tomato, avocado, red onion, lemon juice, lime juice, cilantro, salt, and serrano chile (optional), and stir to combine.

Marinate for 10-15 minutes.

Spoon the shrimp mixture onto the tostadas.

Enjoy!

Ham & Cheese Chicken Rollups

Things You Need

for 4 servings

2 boneless, skinless chicken breasts

1 teaspoon salt, for chicken

¼ teaspoon pepper, for chicken

1 teaspoon garlic powder

4 slices ham

4 slices provolone cheese

1 cup flour (125 g)

2 eggs, beaten

1 cup breadcrumb (115 g)

3 cups broccoli floret (450 g)

4 tablespoons olive oil

1 teaspoon salt

¼ teaspoon pepper

Instructions

Preheat oven to 400°F (200°C)

Cut about ¾ of the way through the chicken horizontally, making sure not to cut through the other side. Flip the chicken open and flat.

Lay a sheet of plastic wrap on top of the chicken and pound it flatter using a pot or a pan. Remove the plastic wrap.

Season with the salt, pepper, and garlic powder, rubbing the seasoning in evenly. Lay 2-3 slices of ham over the chicken, followed by 4 slices of provolone cheese.

Carefully roll the chicken up.

Transfer the flour, eggs, and breadcrumbs into 3 separate bowls.

Dip the chicken roll into the flour, tapping off any excess, and then into the egg, followed by the breadcrumbs. Place on a baking sheet

Add the broccoli to the baking sheet, mixing it with the olive oil, salt, and pepper. Make sure to save a little oil to drizzle on top of the chicken.

Bake for 20 minutes.

Slice, then serve!

Enjoy!

Protein-Packed Chili

Things You Need

for 8 servings

1 tablespoon oil

8 cloves garlic, minced

1 onion, chopped

1 red bell pepper, chopped

1 jalapeño, chopped, seeded

1 teaspoon salt, to taste

¼ teaspoon pepper, to taste

1 tablespoon cayenne pepper

4 tablespoons chili powder

1 tablespoon cumin

4 tomatoes, cubed

28 oz crushed tomato (795 g), 1 can

4 cups vegetable broth (960 mL)

2 cups water (480 mL)

1 ½ cups q uinoa (255 g), rinsed

1 cup red kidney bean (175 g), drained

1 cup pinto bean (175 g), drained

1 cup black beans (170 g), drained

1 cup corn (175 g), fresh or frozen

1 tablespoon lime juice

1 teaspoon dried oregano

1 tablespoon fresh cilantro

avocado, for garnish

Instructions

In a large pot, over medium heat, combine oil, garlic, onion, pepper, jalapeño, salt, pepper, cayenne pepper, chili powder, and cumin. Sauté until onion is translucent, 5-6 minutes.

Add tomatoes, crushed tomatoes, vegetable broth, water, q uinoa, kidney beans, pinto beans, and black beans. Bring to a boil.

Cover and reduce to a simmer for 25-30 minutes.

Add corn, lime juice, oregano, and cilantro, cover again and simmer for 5 minutes.

Allow to cool 2 minutes. Serve topped with avocado and cilantro.

Enjoy!

Tortilla Bowl Southwestern Salad

Things You Need

for 4 servings

4 teaspoons vegetable oil

4 large flour tortillas

2 romaine lettuce hearts

2 tomatoes

½ red onion

2 avocados

1 cup corn (175 g), canned, rinsed and drained

1 cup black beans (170 g), canned, rinsed and drained

¼ cup olive oil (60 mL)

¼ cup lime juice (60 mL)

1 clove garlic, minced

⅛ teaspoon cumin

½ teaspoon red pepper flakes

3 tablespoons fresh cilantro, chopped

½ teaspoon salt

½ teaspoon pepper

Instructions

Preheat the oven to 350°F (180°C).

Pour the vegetable oil (1 teaspoon per bowl) into medium (1.2 q uart) oven-proof bowls and rub around to coat the surface. Press each tortilla into a greased bowl.

Bake for about 10 minutes, until golden brown. Let the tortilla bowls cool.

Make 3 cuts lengthwise on each of the romaine hearts, remove the stems, and chop into smaller pieces. Rinse, drain, and place in a large salad bowl.

Dice the tomatoes and add them to the bowl with the romaine.

Dice the onion and add it to the salad.

Cut the avocados in half, remove the pits, and dice. Add to the salad.

Add the corn and black beans.

In a small bowl or liquid measuring cup, combine the olive oil, lime juice, garlic, cumin, red pepper flakes, cilantro, salt, and pepper. Mix well.

Pour the dressing over the salad and toss well.

Fill each tortilla bowl with the salad.

Enjoy!

Cilantro Lime Chicken & Veggie Rice Meal Prep

Things You Need

for 4 servings

oil, of your preference, to taste

1 lb boneless, skinless chicken breast (455 g), cubed

salt, to taste

pepper, to taste

1 lime, juiced

⅓ cup fresh cilantro (15 g), minced

1 red bell pepper, diced

½ red onion, diced

2 cloves garlic, minced

1 bag riced cauliflower

1 cup corn (175 g), steamed

½ teaspoon chili powder, optional

1 can black beans, rinsed and drained, optional

lime, cut into wedges, optional

Instructions

Heat preferred cooking oil in a large skillet over medium-high heat. Add chicken, season with salt and pepper, and cook until cooked through and no longer pink.

Add lime juice and cilantro. Stir to combine. Remove chicken from pan, place on a plate, and set aside.

Add a little more oil to pan if needed, then add red onion, bell pepper, and garlic. Stir to combine. Allow to cook until onion begins to turn transparent, stirring occasionally.

Add riced cauliflower, corn, and chili powder. Cook until cauliflower is soft and remove from heat.

Distribute black beans, chicken, and cauliflower mixture evenly between 4 containers. Top with a wedge of lime.

This meal prep can be refrigerated for up to 4 days.

Enjoy!

Elevated Hamburger Helper

Things You Need

for 4 servings

8 oz bacon (225 g), chopped

1 small yellow onion, chopped

½ cup red bell pepper (50 g), minced

1 cup shredded carrot (100 g)

2 cloves garlic, grated

1 lb lean ground beef (425 g)

kosher salt, to taste

1 tablespoon smoked paprika

2 tablespoons tomato paste, preferable double-concentrated

1 can diced tomato, petite

3 cups beef stock (720 mL)

2 cups whole milk (480 mL)

1 lb pasta shells (425 g), or short noodles of choice

2 cups shredded smoked gouda cheese (200 g)

2 cups shredded cheddar cheese (200 g)

fresh parsley, for garnish

Instructions

Add the bacon to a large pot. Turn the heat to medium-high and cook until crispy, 5–7 minutes. Using a slotted spoon, transfer the bacon to a paper towel-lined plate to drain. Discard all but 1 tablespoon of the rendered bacon fat in the pot.

Reduce the heat to medium and add the onion to the pot. Cook until softened, 5–7 minutes. Add the red bell pepper, carrots, and garlic. Cook until softened, 2–3 minutes more.

Increase the heat to medium-high and add the ground beef to the pan. Break up the beef with spatula and cook until browned, about 5 minutes. Season with salt.

Add the paprika and tomato paste. Cook until fragrant and the tomato paste turns brick-red in color, 2–3 minutes. Add the diced tomatoes, beef stock, and milk and bring to a low boil.

Once the liquid is boiling, add the pasta shells. Cover and cook for about 10 minutes, stirring occasionally, until the noodles are al dente and they have absorbed most of the liq uid. NOTE: The timing will differ depending on what type of noodles you use.

Remove the pot from the heat. Stir in the Gouda and cheddar cheeses until melted. Fold in the cooked bacon.

Garnish with parsley, if desired.

Serve immediately.

Enjoy!

Chicken Tortilla Soup

Things You Need

for 1 serving

1 tablespoon cooking oil, of preference

1 clove garlic, minced

2 tablespoons white onion, diced

¼ cup tomato (50 g), diced

1 tablespoon green chilli, diced

¼ cup black beans (40 g)

¼ cup frozen corn (45 g)

salt, to taste

pepper, to taste

⅛ teaspoon dried oregano

⅛ teaspoon cumin

⅛ teaspoon chili powder

1 ½ cups chicken broth (355 mL), or veggie broth

1 cup rotisserie chicken (125 g), shredded

tortilla strip, for Garnish

fresh cilantro, for Garnish

Instructions

In a medium sauce pot over a medium heat, add oil, garlic and onion. Cook until onion starts to become translucent.

Add tomatoes, green chiles, black beans, corn, salt, pepper, oregano, cumin, and chili powder. Cook until all ingredients are heated through, stirring occasionally.

Add broth, stir and bring to a simmer.

Add chicken and allow to heat through.

Serve with a sprinkle of tortilla strips and cilantro.

Enjoy!

One-pan Chicken Sausage & Veggies

Things You Need

for 4 servings

1 zucchini, sliced

1 yellow sq uash, sliced

1 tablespoon olive oil

¼ teaspoon salt

¼ teaspoon pepper

¼ teaspoon garlic powder

4 chicken sausages, fully cooked, sliced

4 cups wild rice (920 g), cooked, to serve

Instructions

Preheat the oven to 400°F (200°C).

Place the sq uash and zucchini on a baking sheet. Evenly coat with olive oil, salt, pepper, and garlic powder.

Push the sq uash and zucchini to the sides and place the chicken sausage in the middle.

Bake for 15 minutes, or until the zucchini and squash are tender.

Serve with wild rice. Eat immediately or refrigerate in airtight container up to 3-4 days.

Enjoy!

Sweet Potato And Black Bean Burritos

Things You Need

for 3 servings

2 medium sweet potatoes, peeled and cubed

olive oil, to taste

½ teaspoon smoked paprika

½ teaspoon garlic powder

kosher salt, to taste

pepper, to taste

½ medium yellow onion, diced

1 jalapeño, seeded and diced

1 clove garlic, minced

1 teaspoon chili powder

½ teaspoon ground cumin

cayenne pepper, to taste

15 oz black beans (425 g), 1 can, drained and rinsed

¾ cup corn (130 g)

3 large flour tortillas

lettuce, chopped, for serving

diced tomato, for serving

shredded vegan cheddar cheese, for serving

guacamole, for serving

Instructions

Preheat the oven to 400°F (200°C).

Add the sweet potatoes to a baking sheet with a drizzle of olive oil, the paprika, garlic powder, salt, and pepper. Toss until well coated.

Bake for 20 minutes, flipping halfway through, until the sweet potato is tender.

Heat a drizzle of olive oil in a large saucepan over medium heat. Once the oil begins to shimmer, add the onion and cook for 3-4 minutes, until semi-translucent. Add the jalapeño, garlic, chili powder, cumin, and cayenne pepper and cook for 2-3 minutes, until the spices are fragrant. Add the black beans and corn, season with salt and pepper, and cook until warmed through, 3-4 more minutes.

To assemble a burrito, add ⅓ of the bean and corn mixture, ⅓ of the roasted sweet potatoes, some lettuce, tomatoes, vegan cheese, and guacamole to the center of a tortilla. Fold in the sides and roll up, keeping the filling tucked in place. Repeat with the remaining Things You Need. Cut in half and serve.

Enjoy!

Chicken Enchilada-Stuffed Zucchini Boats

Things You Need

for 1 serving

1 boneless, skinless chicken breast, sliced into ½-inch (1 cm) pieces

½ teaspoon salt

¼ teaspoon ground black pepper

½ teaspoon chili powder

2 teaspoons olive oil

½ cup salsa (130 g), mild

1 zucchini, cut in half lengthwise, centers hollowed out

2 tablespoons shredded cheddar cheese

1 roma tomato, diced

¼ avocado, dinced

2 tablespoons chopped cilantro

1 lime, cut into wedges

Lime Crema

½ cup nonfat greek yogurt (140 g), plain

1 tablespoon lime juice

¼ teaspoon salt

Instructions

Preheat oven to 375°F (190°C).

Cut zucchini in half and hollow out the centers

Add the Greek yogurt, lime juice, and salt together in a small bowl and stir to combine.

On a cutting board, season the chicken breast with salt, pepper, and chili powder.

Heat olive oil in a large pan over medium heat. Once the oil begins to shimmer, add the chicken and cook until browned, about 3 minutes.

Remove the chicken from the pan and let cool. Once cooled, shred the chicken with a fork.

Add the chicken to a bowl with the salsa and stir to combine.

Stuff chicken mixture in hollowed out zucchini boats, and top with cheddar cheese.

Bake until cheese is melted and browned, and zucchini is tender, about 20 minutes.

Top with tomato, avocado, cilantro, and lime crema. Serve with lime wedges.

Enjoy!

Tofu Stir Fry

Things You Need

for 2 servings

4 cloves garlic, minced, divided

2 teaspoons fresh ginger, grated

1 tablespoon honey

1 teaspoon sriracha

¼ cup lime juice (60 mL)

¼ cup reduced sodium soy sauce (60 mL)

1 block extra firm tofu

2 tablespoons sesame oil

1 cup sliced white onion

1 cup sliced carrot

1 cup sliced red bell pepper

½ cup edamame (75 g), frozen, thawed

3 cups soba noodle (300 g), cooked

1 tablespoon sesame seed

green onion, chopped, to serve

Instructions

In a medium bowl, mix together 2 cloves of garlic, the ginger, honey, Sriracha, lime juice, and soy sauce. Set aside.

Wrap the tofu in a dish towel, then place a plate on top. Let drain for 10-15 minutes, then remove the plate, unwrap the tofu, and slice into cubes.

In a wok or large frying pan, heat the sesame oil over medium heat. Add the tofu and pan fry for 5-7 minutes, stirring occasionally.

Add the remaining 2 cloves of minced garlic and the onion and stir until softened, about 1 minute.

Add the carrot, bell pepper, and edamame and cook, stirring occasionally, until tender, 2-3 minutes.

Add the soba noodles, reserved sauce, and sesame seeds. Cook for 1-2 minutes, stirring occasionally, until warmed through. Remove the pan from the heat.

Garnish with green onions, if desired.

Enjoy!

Eggplant Parmesan Boats

Things You Need

for 4 servings

2 medium eggplants

2 tablespoons olive oil

salt, to taste

pepper, to taste

½ lb ground turkey (225 g)

1 onion, diced

2 cups marinara sauce (520 g)

2 cloves garlic, minced

1 cup shredded low-fat mozzarella (100 g)

½ cup grated parmesan cheese (55 g)

fresh basil, for Garnish

Instructions

Preheat oven to 400°F (200°C).

Scoop out inside of eggplant leaving about ½-inch (1 cm) border inside.

Chop the remaining eggplant and reserve.

Brush the scooped out eggplants with olive oil, sprinkle with salt and pepper.

Bake for 10-15 minutes.

Heat olive oil in medium skillet over medium heat.

Add onions and garlic to the pan. Cook until translucent. Add ground turkey and season with garlic powder, salt and pepper. Cook until the meat is browned.

Add leftover eggplant pieces to ground turkey and onion. Cook for 5-8 minutes or until tender.

Add marinara sauce and cook for another 3-5 minutes.

Scoop meat sauce into the eggplants and sprinkle with mozzarella and parmesan.

Bake for 10-15 minutes, or until cheese is melted.

Sprinkle with basil and serve.

Enjoy!

ANTI-COLITIS DINNER RECIPES

Keto Friendly Spinach & Artichoke Chicken Rolls

Things You Need

for 4 servings

2 cloves garlic, minced

10 oz spinach (285 g)

1 cup artichoke heart (170 g), chopped

2 oz cream cheese (55 g), softened

½ cup shredded mozzarella cheese (50 g)

⅔ cup grated parmesan cheese (75 g)

salt, to taste

pepper, to taste

4 boneless, skinless chicken breasts

1 teaspoon salt

1 teaspoon pepper

½ teaspoon onion powder

½ teaspoon garlic powder

1 ⅓ cups riced cauliflower (135 g), to serve

2 cups broccoli (300 g), cooked, to serve

Instructions

Add a tablespoon of olive oil to a skillet over medium-high heat. Once the oil begins to shimmer, add garlic and cook for 30 seconds, stirring constantly.

Add the spinach and artichoke, and stir.

Mix in cream cheese, mozzarella, and Parmesan cheese, and stir until the cheeses are well incorporated. Remove from the heat and set aside.

Preheat oven to 400°F (200°C).

Sprinkle the chicken breasts with salt, pepper, onion powder, and garlic powder until evenly coated.

To pound out the chicken, take a chicken breast and butterfly it by slicing half way into it to open like a book, making sure not to slice all the way through. Cover the breast with parchment paper or plastic wrap. Gently pound the meat with a mallet or rolling pin until it is evenly flattened, about ¼ inch (6 mm) in thickness.

Onto each pounded chicken breast, evenly add ¼ of the spinach-artichoke mixture, but making sure to not overfill the chicken.

Carefully roll the chicken breast until the ends overlap and then place the chicken into a greased baking dish.

Bake for 20 minutes or until the chicken is fully opaque and reaches at least 165°F (75°C).

Serve with riced cauliflower, broccoli, or other low carb vegetables of your choice.

Eat right away or refrigerate until ready to eat.

Enjoy!

Chorizo Tomato Rotini Pasta

Things You Need

for 3 servings

1 tablespoon oil

4 oz chorizo (110 g), chopped

½ onion, chopped

1 lb ground beef (455 g)

2 teaspoons salt

2 teaspoons pepper

3 cups tomato sauce (450 g)

1 ¼ cups rotini pasta (250 g)

½ cup parmesan cheese (50 g)

½ cup fresh basil (12 g), chopped

Instructions

Heat oil in a large pot over medium-high heat.

Cook chorizo until slightly crispy.

Add the onions and cook until translucent.

Add the beef, salt, and pepper, cooking until no pink is showing.

Pour in the tomato sauce, and cook until sauce thickens.

Add the pasta, parmesan, and basil, stirring until the pasta is evenly coated.

Enjoy!

Garlic Veggie Rotini Pasta

Things You Need

for 3 servings

2 tablespoons oil

2 cups mushrooms (150 g), sliced

2 cups broccoli (500 g), chopped

4 cloves garlic, chopped

2 bell peppers, sliced

1 tablespoon dried oregano

2 teaspoons salt

2 teaspoons pepper

1 ¼ cups rotini pasta (250 g)

Instructions

Heat oil in a large pot over high heat.

Cook mushrooms, broccoli, garlic, peppers, oregano, salt, and pepper until the vegetables are tender.

Add in the pasta and stir until evenly mixed.

Enjoy!

Sausage, Spinach, Tomato Rigatoni

Things You Need

for 6 servings

1 tablespoon olive oil

5 links hot italian sausage

1 large yellow onion, chopped

5 cloves garlic, minced

salt, to taste

pepper, to taste

1 tablespoon dried oregano

1 tablespoon dried basil

1 tablespoon dried parsley

12 oz tomato paste (340 g)

15 oz diced tomato (425 g)

2 cups grated parmesan cheese (220 g), divided

2 cups spinach (80 g)

1 lb rigatoni (455 g), cooked

1 cup ricotta cheese (245 g)

fresh basil, to Garnish

Instructions

To a large dutch oven on medium heat, add the olive oil and heat it until it shimmers.

Add the hot Italian sausage, cook until the the first side browns deeply, flip and cook on the other side until the sausage is fully cooked, 15 minutes. Remove the sausages from the pan and slice when they cool down.

To the leftover pan drippings, add the chopped yellow onion, minced garlic, salt, pepper, dried basil, dried oregano, and dried parsley. Cook until the onions are caramelized and soft. About 10 minutes.

Add the tomato paste and cook until the tomato paste darkens slightly.

Add in the diced tomatoes and the sausage slices into the pan, stir, and let the sauce come to a simmer.

Add in half the grated parmesan, spinach, the cooked pasta, and stir to combine.

Spoon in fresh dollaps of the ricotta cheese, Garnish with fresh basil, more grated parmesan, and serve!

Enjoy!

Slow Cooker Balsamic Chicken

Things You Need

for 4 servings

1 tablespoon olive oil

4 cloves garlic, minced

1 lb baby carrot (455 g)

8 boneless, skinless chicken thighs

1 teaspoon salt

1 teaspoon pepper

1 teaspoon garlic powder

1 teaspoon dried basil

½ cup balsamic vinegar (120 mL)

1 onion, sliced

1 lb green beans (455 g)

fresh parsley, chopped, for Garnish

Instructions

Pour olive oil and garlic in the bottom of a 6-qt slow cooker. Line the bottom with baby carrots, then place the chicken thighs over the carrots.

Season the chicken thighs with salt, pepper, garlic powder, basil and vinegar. Top with sliced onion.

Cover and cook on low heat for 8 hours or high for 4 hours. Add green beans during the last 30 minutes of cooking time.

Sprinkle with fresh chopped parsley and serve immediately.

Enjoy!

Tomato And Anchovy Pasta

Things You Need

for 4 servings

1 tablespoon unsalted butter

10 anchovies, finely chopped, divided

½ cup panko breadcrumbs (25 g)

½ cup freshly grated parmigiano-reggiano cheese (55 g)

¼ cup extra virgin olive oil (60 mL), plus 1 tablespoon, divided

6 cloves garlic, minced

½ teaspoon red pepper flakes

2 pt cherry tomato (400 g), halved

1 teaspoon kosher salt, plus more to taste

1 cup white wine (240 mL)

1 lb spaghetti (455 g), cooked al dente, 1/4 cup (60 ml) cooking water reserved

lemon zest, to taste

Instructions

Melt the butter in a large skillet over medium heat. Add 4 of the chopped anchovy filets and cook for 1 minute, until they begin to melt.

Add the panko bread crumbs and cook for 3 minutes, stirring freq uently, until golden brown. Transfer the bread crumbs to a medium bowl and let cool to room temperature. Once cooled, toss with the Parmigiano-Reggiano cheese.

Heat ¼ cup (60 ml) of olive oil in a medium saucepan over medium-high heat. Once the oil begins to shimmer, add the remaining 6 anchovies and cook for 2 minutes, stirring freq uently, until the anchovies begin to melt into the oil.

Add the garlic and red pepper flakes and cook for 30 seconds, until fragrant.

Add the tomatoes and stir to coat in the oil. Season with 1 teaspoon of salt and cook for 5 minutes, or until the tomatoes just begin to soften.

Add the white wine and reduce the heat to low. Cook for 5 minutes, or until the sauce is reduced by half.

Add cooked pasta and reserved cooking water to the pot with the tomatoes and stir to combine. Cook for 1 minute, until the pasta is well coated and saucy. Drizzle with the remaining tablespoon of olive oil and season with salt. Toss to coat.

Serve the pasta topped with the anchovy bread crumbs and lemon zest

Enjoy!

Cajun Chicken Alfredo

Things You Need

for 4 servings

3 tablespoons olive oil

3 cloves garlic, chopped

1 cup cooked sausage (140 g), sliced

2 chicken breasts, thinly sliced

1 tablespoon cajun seasoning

2 cups heavy cream (480 mL)

4 cups penne pasta (400 g), cooked

1 cup parmesan cheese (110 g)

¼ cup fresh parsley (10 g)

Instructions

Heat oil in a large pot over high heat. Cook the garlic, sausage, and chicken until garlic starts to brown and the chicken is no longer pink.

Sprinkle over the Cajun seasoning and stir to evenly coat the sausage and chicken.

Add the cream, and bring to a boil.

Add the pasta, stirring until evenly mixed.

To finish, add parmesan and parsley, stirring until cheese melts and pasta is coated with a thick sauce.

Serve.

Enjoy!

Garlic Shrimp Scampi

Things You Need

for 2 servings

3 tablespoons butter

3 cloves garlic, chopped

1 lb shrimp (455 g), peeled and deveined

1 teaspoon salt

1 teaspoon pepper

½ lemon, juiced

1 teaspoon red chili flake

¼ cup fresh parsley (10 g), chopped

½ lb spaghetti (225 g), cooked

Instructions

Heat the pot over medium heat.

Melt the butter in the pot.

Cook the garlic until it starts to brown.

Add the shrimp, salt, and pepper, cooking until shrimp is pink all the way through.

Add the lemon juice, chili flakes, and parsley.

Add the spaghetti, and toss until evenly coated.

Enjoy!

Avocado Lime Salmon

Things You Need

for 1 serving

6 oz skinless salmon (170 g)

1 clove garlic, minced

olive oil, to taste

salt, to taste

pepper, to taste

½ teaspoon paprika

Avocado Topping

1 avocado, chopped

¼ red onion, chopped

1 tablespoon fresh cilantro, chopped

1 tablespoon olive oil

salt, to taste

pepper, to taste

1 tablespoon lime juice

Instructions

Preheat the oven to 400°F (200°C). Line a baking sheet with parchment paper.

On the prepared baking sheet, rub the salmon with the garlic, olive oil, salt, pepper, and paprika.

Bake for 10-12 minutes, until cooked through.

Make the avocado topping: In a small bowl, gently mix together the avocado, red onion, cilantro, olive oil, salt, pepper, and lime juice. Don't overmix or you'll break down the avocado.

Spoon the avocado topping over the salmon.

Enjoy!

Fajita Pasta Bake

Things You Need

for 6 servings

1 yellow bell pepper, seeded and sliced

1 green bell pepper, seeded and sliced

1 red bell pepper, seeded and sliced

2 ½ cups mushroom (185 g), sliced

1 medium yellow onion, diced

1 tablespoon chili powder

1 tablespoon paprika

1 tablespoon garlic powder

1 tablespoon cumin

1 teaspoon salt

1 teaspoon pepper

3 tablespoons olive oil

4 cups penne pasta (400 g), uncooked

1 ½ cups sour cream (345 g)

3 cups shredded pepper jack cheese (300 g)

fresh parsley, chopped. for Garnish

Instructions

Preheat the oven to 400°F (200°C).

In a nonstick baking dish, add the bell peppers, mushrooms, and onion.

In a small bowl, combine the chili powder, paprika, garlic powder, cumin, salt, and pepper.

Pour the olive oil and half of the spice mix over the vegetables and toss well to coat.

Bake the vegetables for about 30 minutes, stirring occasionally, until tender.

In a large pot of boiling water, cook the pasta according to the package instructions, until tender.

Drain the pasta, reserving about 1 cup (240 ml) of cooking water.

Return the drained pasta to the pot and add the roasted vegetables. Add the rest of the spice mix, the reserved pasta water, and the sour cream and mix to combine.

Transfer the pasta mixture to the baking dish used for roasting the vegetables and spread evenly. Sprinkle the cheese over the top.

Bake for about 15 minutes, until the cheese is golden brown.

Let cool for about 5 minutes, then serve. Garnish with parsley, if desired.

Enjoy!

Spaghetti With Fresh Tomato Sauce

Things You Need

for 4 servings

1 lb spaghetti (455 g)

2 tablespoons olive oil

3 cloves garlic, minced

2 cups cherry tomato (400 g)

salt, to taste

pepper, to taste

1 cup white wine (235 mL)

1 cup parmesan cheese (110 g)

½ cup fresh basil (20 g), chopped

Instructions

Cook spaghetti in boiling salted water until it's al dente. Reserve 1 cup (235 ml) of the pasta water before draining.

While the spaghetti is cooking, heat olive oil in a large pan (it should be large enough to toss the pasta in). Add garlic and tomatoes, and stir until well-incorporated. Season with salt and pepper.

Cook tomatoes down for 5 minutes until they soften and release some of their juices.

Then add the wine and allow that to reduce for 5-10 minutes until you're left with a syrupy sauce.

Add the pasta to your sauce, along with a splash of pasta water and toss to coat it for about 1-2 minutes so the pasta finishes cooking and absorbs the flavor of the sauce.

Add the parmesan and basil. Add another small splash of pasta water, if needed. Toss until the cheese is melted down and you're left with a smooth sauce.

Gradually add small amounts of pasta water, as needed, until the sauce reaches your desired smoothness.

Top off with extra parmesan and basil and serve immediately.

Enjoy!

Loaded Baked Potato Soup

Things You Need

for 6 servings

4 lb russet potato (1.8 g), washed

1 tablespoon olive oil

1 teaspoon salt

½ teaspoon pepper

1 onion, diced

3 cloves garlic

3 tablespoons butter

¼ cup flour (30 g)

2 ½ cups chicken broth (590 mL)

8 oz cream cheese (225 g)

Garnish

shredded cheese

bacon, diced

fresh chive, chopped

Instructions

Preheat your oven to 425°F (220°C).

On a parchment paper-lined baking sheet, rub potatoes with salt, pepper, and olive oil.

Bake in preheated oven for 40-50 minutes.

Once cooled, peel and mash potatoes, and set aside.

Heat oil in large pot over a medium-high heat.

Add onion and garlic. Cook until translucent and garlic is fragant, about 5 minutes.

Add butter and melt.

Bring in flour and stir until mixture is lightly browned.

Add in the chicken broth and cream cheese. Stir until fully incorporated

Add in the mashed potatoes and combine.

Season with salt and pepper.

Garnish bowl with shredded cheese, bacon, and chives.

Enjoy!

Cashew Chicken Stir-Fry

Things You Need

for 4 servings

6 tablespoons soy sauce

1 tablespoon hoisin sauce

1 tablespoon rice vinegar

2 tablespoons honey

1 teaspoon sesame oil

½ tablespoon ginger, minced

2 cloves garlic, minced

¾ lb chicken breast (340 g), cut into 1-inch (2 1/2 cm) pieces

salt, to taste

pepper, to taste

1 tablespoon cornstarch

1 tablespoon sesame oil

4 cups broccoli floret (600 g)

1 red bell pepper, cut into 1-inch (2 1/2 cm) pieces

¾ cup raw cashew (95 g)

½ cup water (120 mL)

brown rice, to serve

Instructions

In a medium bowl, combine the soy sauce, hoisin sauce, rice vinegar, honey, sesame oil, ginger, and garlic. Set aside.

In a medium bowl, season the chicken with salt, pepper, and cornstarch.

Heat a 9.5" fry pan over medium-high heat and add sesame oil.

Add the chicken and cook for 5-6 minutes, or until the chicken begins to brown.

Remove chicken and set aside in a separate bowl.

Add the broccoli and bell peppers, and cook for 2-3 minutes.

Add the chicken, cashews and sauce. Stir together and allow sauce to thicken.

Remove from heat and serve over brown rice.

Enjoy!

Avocado Quinoa Power Salad

Things You Need

for 6 servings

Salad

2 cups water (480 mL)

salt, to taste

1 cup q uinoa (170 g), rinsed

2 cups fresh spinach (80 g), roughly chopped

1 large cucumber, diced

4 roma tomatoes, diced

2 ripe avocados, pits removed and diced

1 lemon, juiced

4 tablespoons extra virgin olive oil

pepper, to taste

Instructions

In a small saucepan, bring the water and a pinch of salt to a boil. Add the quinoa, cover, and simmer for 15 minutes, or until the water is absorbed. Transfer to a medium bowl to cool to room temperature, then fluff the quinoa.

Refrigerate the quinoa for 20 minutes.

Add the spinach, cucumber, tomatoes, and avocado to the bowl of q uinoa and mix to combine.

Add the lemon juice, olive oil, salt, and pepper, and mix well.

Enjoy!

One-Pan Chicken And Broccoli Stir Fry

Things You Need

for 2 servings

1 lb chicken (455 g), cubed

1 teaspoon salt

1 teaspoon pepper

1 cup broccoli (150 g), chopped

1 cup bell pepper (100 g), diced

Stir-Fry Sauce

½ cup soy sauce (120 mL)

¼ cup honey (85 g)

2 cloves garlic

1 teaspoon ginger

1 tablespoon sesame seed

Instructions

Mix together all sauce ingredients in a small
bowl.

Heat oil over a nonstick pan and add chicken
stirring until cooked.

Pour sauce in pan and stir to coat meat.

Once the sauce is bubbling, add the veggies to
the pan and stir again to coat.

Cook until meat is cooked through and veggies are soft.

Serve over rice or alone.

Enjoy!

Tomato Basil Sausage Spaghetti

Things You Need

for 2 servings

½ lb ground sausage (225 g)

½ onion, diced

1 teaspoon salt

1 teaspoon pepper

2 cups marinara sauce (500 g)

1 cup milk (240 mL)

½ cup fresh basil (20 g), chopped

½ lb spaghetti (225 g), cooked

Instructions

Heat pot to medium-high heat.

Cook the sausage in the pot.

Add the onions, salt, and pepper, cooking until the onions are translucent and sausage is starting to brown.

Add the marinara, milk, and basil, cooking until sauce has thickened slightly.

Add the spaghetti, and toss until evenly coated and sauce sticks to the noodles.

Enjoy!

Easy Chickpea Curry (Channa Masala)

Things You Need

for 4 servings

1 tablespoon vegetable oil

1 large onion, diced

2 cloves garlic, minced

ginger, peeled and grated, 1 inch (2 1/2 cm) piece

1 jalapeño, or green chile, seeded and sliced

2 tablespoons garam masala

1 teaspoon turmeric

1 teaspoon salt

1 teaspoon black pepper

2 cups fresh tomato (400 g), diced

15 oz chickpeas (425 g), drained and rinsed, 2 cans

½ cup water (120 mL)

½ lemon, juiced

¼ cup fresh cilantro (10 g), chopped

Instructions

Heat olive oil in a large stock pot or dutch oven over medium-high heat.

Add onion and cook until onion becomes translucent and begins to brown, about 3-5 minutes.

Add garlic, ginger, and jalapeño. Continue to cook over medium heat until garlic is fragrant and jalapeño is tender, about 3-4 minutes.

Add garam masala, turmeric, salt, and pepper then continue to cook for 1-2 minutes.

Add tomatoes, chickpeas, and water. Stir to incorporate, making sure to use the spoon the scrape off any brown bits that have appeared on the bottom or sides of the pot.

As the tomatoes break down, the mixture should take on the texture of a thick stew. Add more water if needed before bringing everything to a simmer and then cover with a lid.

Once covered, cook for 15 minutes while stirring occasionally.

Remove lid, reduce heat to low and mix in the lemon juice and chopped cilantro. Cook over low heat 1-2 minutes until the cilantro has wilted and turned bright green.

Serve over basmati rice or with a side of naan.

Enjoy!

Spinach Mushroom Pesto Spaghetti

Things You Need

for 2 servings

1 tablespoon canola oil

5 oz spinach (140 g)

2 cups mushroom (150 g), sliced

1 teaspoon salt

1 teaspoon pepper

1 cup pesto (225 g)

½ cup parmesan cheese (110 g)

½ lb spaghetti (225 g), cooked

Instructions

Heat pot over medium-high heat.

Add oil to the pot.

Cook the spinach until wilted.

Add the mushrooms, salt, and pepper cooking
until most of the water is gone.

Add the pesto and parmesan.

Add the spaghetti, and toss until evenly coated,
with the sauce sticking to the noodles.

Enjoy!

Easy-Peasy Potato Curry

Things You Need

for 4 servings

2 tablespoons vegetable oil

1 medium yellow onion, diced

4 cloves garlic, minced

4 teaspoons curry powder

1 ½ teaspoons paprika

1 teaspoon cayenne

2 teaspoons cumin powder

½ teaspoon allspice

2 teaspoons fresh ginger, minced

½ teaspoon black pepper

2 lb potato (905 g), peeled and cubed

15 oz chickpeas (425 g), 1 can, drained

1 cup vegetable broth (240 mL)

1 tablespoon lemon juice

14 oz diced tomato (395 g), 1 can

14 oz coconut milk (415 mL), 1 can

rice, cooked, for serving

naan bread, for serving

fresh cilantro, chopped, for garnish

Instructions

Heat the oil in a large pot over medium heat until shimmering. Add the onion and saute for about 3 minutes, until translucent.

Add the garlic and saute for about 2 minutes, until fragrant.

Add the curry powder, paprika, cayenne, cumin, allspice, ginger, salt, and pepper. Stir and cook for about 2 minutes until the spices are fragrant.

Add the potatoes and mix well until well-coated in spices.

Add the chickpeas and stir to incorporate.

Add the broth, lemon juice, and tomatoes and stir, then pour in the coconut milk and stir to combine.

Increase the heat to high and bring the mixture to a simmer. Once bubbling, reduce the heat to medium and cook for 15-20 minutes, until the potatoes are tender and easily pierced with a fork.

Serve with cooked rice and naan and garnish with fresh cilantro.

Enjoy!

One-pan Roasted Chicken And Sweet Potatoes

Things You Need

for 1 serving

1 small sweet potato, diced

1 lemon, sliced, seeds removed

1 cup green beans (360 g), trimmed

1 tablespoon olive oil

1 tablespoon fresh rosemary, chopped

1 tablespoon fresh thyme, chopped

1 clove garlic, minced

½ teaspoon salt, plus more to season

¼ teaspoon ground black pepper, plus more to season

1 boneless, skinless chicken breast

¼ teaspoon paprika

Instructions

Preheat oven to 375°F (190°C).

Add the sweet potatoes, lemon slices, green beans, olive oil, rosemary, thyme, garlic, salt, and pepper to a large bowl (or parchment paper-lined sheet tray) and toss until fully coated.

Season the chicken breast with salt, pepper, and paprika.

Transfer to a parchment paper-lined sheet tray and place the chicken breast on top of the vegetables (if you tossed your vegetables in a bowl).

Bake until vegetables are tender and chicken is cooked through, about 20 minutes.

Enjoy!

Eggplant Potato Tomato Stew

Things You Need

for 5 servings

4 medium yukon potatoes

2 medium eggplants, chopped

2 red bell peppers, seeded and chopped

5 tablespoons olive oil, divided

1 teaspoon salt, plus more to taste, divided

¾ teaspoon pepper, plus more to taste, divided

1 medium yellow onion, diced

1 tablespoon tomato paste

3 cloves garlic, minced

1 teaspoon smoked paprika

15 oz chickpeas (425 g), 1 can, drained and rinsed

3 medium beefsteak tomatoes, diced

1 ½ cups low sodium vegetable broth (360 mL)

fresh parsley, for serving

Instructions

Preheat the oven to 400°F (200°C).

With a sharp knife, score a ring around each potato, just deep enough to break the skin. Place the potatoes in a medium pot of cold water. Bring to a boil and cook for about 8 minutes, until about halfway cooked.

Drain the potatoes, and rinse with cold water. Peel off the skin.

Cut the potatoes into ½-inch (1 cm) pieces and set aside.

Divide the eggplant and bell peppers between 2 baking sheets and spread in an even layer.

Drizzle with 4 tablespoons of olive oil, and season with salt and pepper to taste. Toss with your hands to coat.

Bake for 25 minutes, flipping halfway through.

Heat the remaining tablespoon of olive oil in a large pot over medium heat. Once the oil begins to shimmer, add the onion and cook for 3-4 minutes, until semi-translucent.

Add the tomato paste and stir until well distributed, then add the garlic, paprika, 1 teaspoon salt, and ¾ teaspoon pepper, and cook for another 2-3 minutes, until fragrant.

Add the potatoes, chickpeas, and tomatoes, and stir to incorporate.

Stir in the vegetable broth and cover. Reduce the heat to low and cook for 20 minutes, until the potatoes are tender.

Add the roasted eggplant and bell pepper, and stir to combine. Cook for another 5-10 minutes, until the tomatoes have mostly broken down.

Ladle into bowls, garnish with parsley, and serve. Or, transfer the stew to resealable containers and store in the fridge for up to 5 days or freezer for up to 3 months.

Enjoy!

Chinese Chicken Curry

Things You Need

for 2 servings

3 tablespoons oil

3 cups chicken (400 g)

1 teaspoon salt

1 teaspoon pepper

1 ⅓ cups onion (200 g), chopped

¾ cup carrot (100 g), chopped

1 cup potato (200 g), chopped

4 ¼ cups water (1 L)

⅔ cup peas (100 g)

⅔ cup curry paste (150 g)

Instructions

Heat up 2 tablespoons of oil on low to medium heat.

Sear the chicken until the outside turns golden brown. Season with salt and pepper.

Take out the chicken, make sure you don't clean the pot or you'd wipe away some deliciousness!

Add another tablespoon of oil, fry the onions, carrots, and potatoes until soften.

Add the chicken back in with the water. Bring to a boil then simmer for 10 minutes with the lid on.

Add in the peas and curry paste, stir well.

Serve with rice.

Enjoy!

Cheesesteak-Stuffed Peppers

Things You Need

for 6 servings

1 lb flank steak (455 g)

1 tablespoon olive oil

1 tablespoon paprika

1 tablespoon garlic powder

1 teaspoon pepper, divided

2 teaspoons salt, divided

2 tablespoons worcestershire sauce

2 tablespoons unsalted butter

3 large white onions, sliced

3 green bell peppers, sliced

6 red bell peppers

15 slices provolone cheese

2 tablespoons fresh parsley, chopped, for garnish

Instructions

Preheat the oven to 400°F (200°C).

Cut the flank steak against the grain into ⅛-inch (3-mm) thick slices.

In a large skillet over medium heat, heat the olive oil, until shimmering. Add the steak, paprika, garlic powder, ½ teaspoon of pepper, 1 teaspoon of salt, and the Worcestershire sauce.

Mix to coat the meat with the spices and cook until the meat is cooked through, about 3 minutes. Transfer the meat a bowl, leaving the juices in the pan. Cover and set aside until ready to use.

Add the butter to the pan with the meat juices. Add the onions and cook until tender and shiny, about 10 minutes. Add the green bell peppers and the remaining ½ teaspoon of pepper and teaspoon of salt, and cook until the onions and peppers are caramelized, about 10 minutes.

Cut the top off of a red bell pepper. Cut around the seed pod, then pull it out of the pepper. Remove any remaining seeds. Repeat with the rest of the peppers.

Cut 9 of the provolone slices in half.

Place the peppers in a 9x13-inch (23x33-cm) baking dish, cut side up. Scoop a bit of steak filling into each pepper, followed by the peppers and onions, then 3 half slices of provolone. Repeat with the rest of the steak, then the rest of the peppers and onions. Place a whole slice of provolone on top of each pepper.

Bake for 30 minutes, until the skin of the peppers is shriveling, and the cheese is golden.

Top with parsley.

Enjoy!

Roasted Eggplant Curry

Things You Need

for 6 servings

3 medium eggplants

¼ cup olive oil (60 mL)

sea salt, to taste

½ teaspoon freshly ground pepper, plus more to taste

¼ cup coconut oil (60 mL)

½ medium white onion, chopped

1 teaspoon chili powder

2 teaspoons ground cardamom

1 teaspoon smoked paprika

1 teaspoon ground coriander

1 tablespoon ground turmeric

3 cloves garlic, minced

1 teaspoon ginger, peeled and minced

3 roma tomatoes, Ripe, Diced, Medium size

15 oz coconut milk (425 mL)

½ cup water (120 mL)

cooked rice, for serving

fresh cilantro, chopped, for serving

Instructions

Preheat the oven to 400°F (200°C).

Slice the tops off the eggplants, then slice them in half lengthwise. Cut each half once more lengthwise. Lay the slices on their flat sides and cut lengthwise into thirds. Finally, slice horizontally to form cubes.

Transfer to a baking sheet, drizzle with the olive oil, salt, and pepper. Bake for 25 minutes, stirring halfway through, until golden brown.

In a large saucepan, heat the coconut oil over high hat. Add the onions, stir for 1 minute, then reduce the heat to medium-low and cook, stirring occasionally, until the onions are golden brown, about 8 minutes.

Stir in the chili powder, cardamom, and smoked paprika. Cook until fragrant, about 1 minute.

Stir in the ground coriander, ½ teaspoon of black pepper, turmeric, garlic, and ginger. Cook for a few minutes more, stirring constantly.

Add the chopped tomatoes, coconut milk, water, and the roasted eggplant.

Bring the curry to a simmer, then reduce to low heat, cover, and simmer for 25 minutes. The sauce should reduce and thicken slightly.

Serve the curry warm over rice, topped with chopped cilantro.

Enjoy!

Penne Alla Vodka Pasta

Things You Need

for 3 servings

2 tablespoons olive oil

1 onion, chopped

1 lb ground beef (455 g)

1 teaspoon salt

1 teaspoon pepper

28 oz crushed tomato (795 g), 1 can

½ cup vodka (120 mL)

½ teaspoon red chili flake

½ cup heavy cream (120 mL)

4 cups penne pasta (400 g)

fresh parsley, to garnish

½ cup Parmesan (110 g), to garnish

Instructions

Heat oil in a large pot over high heat. Cook onion until translucent.

Add beef, salt, and pepper, cooking until all the moisture has evaporated and the beef is browned.

Add crushed tomatoes, vodka, and chili flakes, stirring and cooking until half of the liq uid has evaporated and the sauce has reduced.

Add cream, stirring until evenly incorporated.

Stir in pasta until evenly coated.

Serve with parsley and parmesan.

Enjoy!

One-Pot Spicy Sausage And Broccoli Pasta

Things You Need

for 4 servings

2 tablespoons olive oil

1 lb spicy italian sausage (455 g), casing removed

1 lb broccoli florets (455 g)

½ teaspoon red pepper flakes

1 teaspoon kosher salt

½ teaspoon ground black pepper

1 lb rigatoni (455 g)

4 cups chicken stock (960 mL)

½ cup grated parmesan cheese (60 g), plus more garnish

Instructions

Heat the olive oil in a large Dutch oven or heavy-bottomed pot over medium-high heat. Add the sausage and cook until browned, breaking up with a wooden spoon, about 8 minutes.

Add the broccoli, red pepper flakes, salt, and pepper and stir to combine.

Add the pasta and chicken stock and bring to a boil. Cook for 10–12 minutes, stirring constantly, until the liq uid is absorbed and the pasta is tender. Add the Parmesan and stir to incorporate.

Divide the pasta between serving bowls and garnish with more Parmesan.

Enjoy!

Crispy Fish Tacos

Things You Need

for 6 servings

Cabbage Slaw

½ head green cabbage, finely shredded

½ medium red onion, small diced

2 roma tomatoes, diced

¼ cup fresh cilantro (10 g), chopped

1 small jalapeño, diced

2 tablespoons lime juice

salt, to taste

Crispy Fish

1 cup all-purpose flour (125 g)

1 tablespoon old bay seasoning

½ teaspoon baking powder

1 cup lager beer (240 mL)

vegetable oil, for frying

1 lb fresh cod (455 g), cut into 1-inch (2-cm) thick strips

Avocado Crema

2 medium avocados

1 cup sour cream (230 g)

¼ cup lime juice (60 mL)

salt, to taste

Assembly

corn tortilla, warmed

radish, thinly sliced, for serving, optional

Instructions

Make the cabbage slaw: Combine the cabbage, onion, tomato, cilantro, jalapeño, lime juice, and salt in a large bowl. Toss well, then set aside.

Make the crispy fish: In a large bowl, combine the flour, Old Bay, and baking powder. Add the beer and whisk until smooth. Let sit for 15 minutes.

Heat the vegetable oil in a large pot until it reaches 350°F (180°C).

Coat the fish in the batter, then transfer to the oil and fry until golden on the outside and cooked through, 5-7 minutes. Drain the fish on a wire rack set over a baking sheet lined with paper towels.

Make the avocado crema: Add the avocados, sour cream, lime juice, and salt to a blender and blend until smooth.

To assemble the tacos, add a bit of the cabbage slaw to a warmed tortilla. Top with a piece of fried fish, avocado crema, and sliced radish.

Enjoy!

Sesame Peanut Noodles

Things You Need

for 4 servings

½ cup peanut butter (120 g)

3 tablespoons low sodium soy sauce

2 tablespoons sesame oil

2 tablespoons rice vinegar

3 tablespoons water

2 ½ teaspoons brown sugar

1 clove garlic

½ tablespoon fresh ginger, minced

8 oz spaghetti (240 g), cooked according to package instructions

½ cup shredded carrot (55 g)

½ cup shredded red cabbage (50 g)

¾ cup edamame (115 g), shelled

peanut, for garnish

1 tablespoon black sesame seeds, for garnish

scallion, sliced, for garnish

Instructions

In a blender, combine the peanut butter, soy sauce, sesame oil, rice vinegar, water, brown sugar, garlic, and ginger and blend until smooth.

In a large bowl, add the spaghetti, carrots, cabbage, and edamame and pour over the peanut sauce. Use tongs to mix well, until sauce is fully incorporated.

Transfer to bowls and top with peanuts, black sesame seeds, and scallion.

Enjoy!

Garlic Chicken Primavera

Things You Need

for 4 servings

2 tablespoons olive oil

3 cloves garlic, chopped

2 chicken breasts, thinly sliced

2 cups asparagus (250 g), chopped

1 cup cherry tomato (200 g), halved

1 cup carrot (120 g), sliced

1 teaspoon pepper

1 teaspoon salt

4 cups penne pasta (400 g)

1 cup parmesan cheese (110 g)

Instructions

Heat oil in a large pot over high heat. Cook garlic and chicken until no pink is showing.

Add asparagus, tomatoes, carrots, salt, and pepper, cooking for about 2 minutes.

Add pasta and parmesan, stirring until cheese is melted and evenly distributed.

Serve.

Enjoy!

One Pot Chicken Fajita Pasta

Things You Need

for 4 servings

3 tablespoons oil

3 chicken breasts, sliced

1 red bell pepper, sliced

1 green bell pepper, sliced

1 yellow bell pepper, sliced

1 onion, sliced

1 teaspoon salt

1 teaspoon pepper

1 tablespoon chili powder

1 tablespoon cumin

1 tablespoon garlic powder

5 cups milk (1 ¼ L)

4 cups penne pasta (400 g)

1 cup pepper jack cheese (100 g), shredded

Instructions

Heat oil in a large pot over high heat

Add chicken and cook until no pink is visible, about 5-6 minutes, then take the chicken out.

Add the bell peppers and onion, cooking until the onion is translucent, about 6 minutes.

Add the chicken back to the pot with salt, pepper, chili powder, cumin, and garlic powder, stirring until evenly coated, about 30 seconds.

Add the milk and the penne, stirring constantly to prevent any pasta from sticking.

Cook for about 20 minutes until pasta is cooked and the milk has reduced to a thick sauce that coats the pasta.

Add the cheese and mix until melted.

Enjoy!

ANTI-COLITIS DESSERT

Chocolate Hazelnut Mug Cakes

Things You Need

for 2 servings

1 cup chocolate hazelnut spread (300 g), divided

2 large eggs

¼ cup all-purpose flour (30 g)

Instructions

In a medium mixing bowl, whisk together ¾ cup (225 g) chocolate hazelnut spread and the eggs.

Fold in the flour.

Evenly distribute into two mugs.

Microwave each mug for 2 minutes.

Cool for 5 minutes.

Frost with remaining chocolate hazelnut spread and serve warm.

Enjoy!

2-Ingredient Chocolate Soufflé

Things You Need

for 1 serving

½ cup chocolate hazelnut spread (150 g)

2 eggs

Instructions

Preheat the oven to 375°F (190°C).

Separate the egg yolks from the egg whites and place into two bowls.

Mix the chocolate hazelnut spread into the bowl with the egg yolks.

In the second bowl, whisk 2 egg whites until stiff peaks form.

Fold ⅓ of the whipped egg whites into the chocolate/egg yolk mixture until fully incorporated. Add the remaining egg whites to the mixture and fold gently, but thoroughly, until the mixture is smooth.

Pour the mixture into a greased ramekin. Clean the rims so the soufflé rises evenly, and bake for 15-17 minutes.

Serve immediately.

Enjoy!

Strawberry Banana Chia Seed Pudding

Things You Need

for 4 servings

1 banana, mashed

½ cup greek yogurt (140 g)

1 cup almond milk (240 mL)

1 teaspoon vanilla extract

¼ cup chia seeds (40 g)

1 cup strawberry (150 g), diced

Toppings

1 banana, sliced

1 handful strawberry, diced

Instructions

Mash the banana in a medium bowl.

Mix the banana and the yogurt together until smooth.

Pour in the almond milk, vanilla extract, chia seeds, and strawberries, and mix until well combined.

Pour the mixture into an airtight container and refrigerate, covered for 4 hours..

Spoon the pudding into desired serving dish and top with sliced bananas and diced strawberries.

Enjoy!

Chocolate Avocado Brownies

Things You Need

for 2 servings

1 ripe avocado, cubed

2 eggs

½ cup honey (170 g)

1 teaspoon vanilla extract

⅔ cup whole wheat flour (75 g)

¼ cup cocoa powder (30 g)

1 teaspoon baking powder

Instructions

Preheat oven to 350°F (175°C).

In a blender or food processor, combine avocado, eggs, honey and vanilla extract. Blend until smooth, scraping down sides as necessary.

In a large bowl, whisk the flour, cocoa powder and baking powder.

Combine the wet and dry mixtures and fold until a batter forms. Pour batter into a greased 8x8 inch baking pan.

Bake for 20-30 minutes. Allow to cool.

Enjoy!

Classic Chocolate Cake

Things You Need

for 8 servings

Chocolate Cake

nonstick cooking spray, for greasing

2 cups all purpose flour (250 g)

1 cup cocoa powder (120 g)

1 teaspoon kosher salt

1 ½ teaspoons baking soda

1 ½ teaspoons baking powder

2 sticks unsalted butter, room temperature

2 cups granulated sugar (400 g)

2 large eggs, room temperature

2 teaspoons vanilla extract

1 ½ cups sour cream (370 g)

Sour Cream Chocolate Frosting

2 sticks unsalted butter, room temperature

1 ½ cups sour cream (370 g)

2 teaspoons vanilla extract

1 pinch kosher salt

2 ¼ cups powdered sugar (245 g)

⅔ cup cocoa powder (80 g)

Instructions

Preheat the oven to 350°F (180°C).

Make the cake: Grease and line 2 8-inch (22 cm) round cake pans with parchment paper.

In a large bowl, whisk together the flour, cocoa powder, salt, baking soda, and baking powder.

In a separate large bowl, cream the butter and sugar with an electric hand mixer on medium-high speed until light and fluffy, about 2 minutes.

Add the eggs, 1 at a time, and beat until fully incorporated.

Add the vanilla and sour cream and stir with a rubber spatula until starting to incorporate, then beat with the hand mixer until fully combined.

Gradually add the dry ingredients to the wet Things You Need, beating between each addition until just combined.

Divide the batter evenly between the prepared pans. Bake for 30 minutes, or until a toothpick inserted in the center of a cake comes out clean. Let cakes cool for 10 minutes in the pans, then invert onto a wire rack and let cool completely.

Make the frosting: Add the butter, sour cream, vanilla, and salt to a large bowl. Beat with an electric hand mixer on medium speed until well combined. Sift in the powdered sugar and cocoa powder and beat until well incorporated and the frosting is smooth.

Place 1 layer of cake on a cake stand or serving platter lined with strips of parchment paper (for easy removal). Spread ¾ cup frosting evenly over the cake. Place the other cake layer on top and use the rest of the frosting to frost the top and sides of the cake.

Slice and serve.

Enjoy!

Iced Oatmeal Cookies

Things You Need

for 8 servings

2 cups old fashioned rolled oat (200 g), pulsed in food processor x10

2 cups flour (250 g)

½ teaspoon baking powder

2 teaspoons cinnamon

½ teaspoon nutmeg

1 cup unsalted butter (230 g), room temperature and softened

½ cup sugar (100 g)

1 cup brown sugar (220 g)

1 teaspoon vanilla extract

2 eggs

½ cup raisin (75 g)

Icing

2 cups powdered sugar (220 g)

1 ½ tablespoons milk

1 tablespoon warm water

Instructions

Preheat oven to 350°F (180°C)

Pulse oats in a food processor or blender 10 times.

Add pulsed oats, flour, baking powder, cinnamon, and nutmeg into a bowl.

In a large bowl, beat softened butter with a hand mixer until creamy, add brown and white sugars, then beat until fluffy. Next beat in vanilla and eggs 1 at a time.

Pour the dry ingredients into the wet Things You Need ⅓ at a time until it's gone and dough forms.

Fold in raisins or chocolate chunks.

Take 1 tablespoon of dough and roll it into a ball. Then flatten into a cookie shape and put on a well-greased parchment-lined baking sheet.

Bake 12-15 minutes. (Top rack = no brown bottoms, bottom rack = browned bottoms and a little more crispy).

Cool completely and make the icing in the meantime. Combine powdered sugar, milk, and warm water in a shallow bowl. Once the cookies have cooled, dip into the icing or dab icing on with a pastry brush. Dry for 10 minutes or until icing has hardened.

Enjoy!

Easiest Banana-cocoa Ice Cream

Things You Need

for 2 servings

4 bananas

1 tablespoon unsweetened cocoa powder, depending on your taste

¼ teaspoon ground cinnamon

strawberry, to garnish

Instructions

Slice bananas and place in an airtight container. Freeze for at least two hours, preferably overnight.

Place frozen banana slices in a food processor and blend until they reach the consistency of soft serve, about 4 minutes.

Add cocoa powder and cinnamon. Blend until just combined.

Serve immediately for soft-serve consistency or transfer to freezer for at least 2 hours for ice cream consistency.

Garnish with strawberries.

Enjoy!

Caramel Rose Apple Pie

Things You Need

for 6 servings

4 apples

1 lemon, juiced

½ cup granulated sugar (100 g)

½ cup brown sugar (110 g)

¼ teaspoon cinnamon

¼ teaspoon nutmeg

1 prepared pie dough

¼ cup heavy cream (60 mL)

Instructions

Peel the apples and place them in a large bowl with enough water to cover. Squeeze lemon juice in the water to prevent the apples from browning. Working with 1 apple at a time, cut around the core, discarding the core and removing the "cheeks." Slice the cheeks very thin.

In a large bowl, combine the granulated sugar, brown sugar, cinnamon and nutmeg. Stir to combine. Add the sliced apples, stir to coat, and let sit for 30 minutes.

Line a pie dough in a 9-inch (23-cm) cast-iron pan, and prick the dough with a fork all around. Chill in the fridge until very firm, 20-30 minutes.

Working in batches, remove the apples from the cinnamon-sugar mixture by taking a handful at a time and carefully sq ueezing them with your hands to remove the excess moisture. Place the drained apples in a separate large bowl, reserving the liq uid to make the caramel sauce.

Preheat the oven to 375°F (190°C).

Working from the outside in, line the apple slices on the pie dough by overlapping each slice to create a rose shape. Roll up 1 apple slice tightly and place it in the center, creating a bud shape. Cover the pan with foil and bake for 30 minutes. Uncover and bake for 10 minutes more, or until golden brown. Remove from the oven and let cool for 10 minutes.

In a saucepan, bring the reserved cinnamon-sugar liquid to a boil. Once the liq uid is reduced by half, 10-15 minutes, add the heavy cream and stir well.

To serve, pour the caramel sauce over the apple pie.

Enjoy!

Classic Chocolate Truffle

Things You Need

for 4 servings

3 cups semi-sweet chocolate chips (525 g)

1 ½ cups heavy cream (360 mL)

Topping

1 cup cocoa powder (120 g)

Instructions

In a medium-sized pan, combine semisweet chocolate chips and heavy cream over low heat, mix until you achieve a smooth consistency.

Pour mixture into a bread pan.

Allow to sit in refrigerator for 1 hour or until mixture is solid.

With an ice cream scoop, form balls from the mixture (refreeze if truffle begins to melt).

Roll in cocoa powder for topping.

Enjoy!

Peanut Butter Banana Crunch Chia Seed Pudding

Things You Need

for 4 servings

½ cup peanut butter (120 g)

½ cup greek yogurt (140 g)

1 cup almond milk (240 mL)

1 teaspoon vanilla extract

2 tablespoons honey

½ cup chia seeds (80 g)

Toppings

1 banana, sliced

roasted peanut

4 tablespoons crunchy granola cluster

Instructions

In a medium bowl, mix the peanut butter and greek yogurt together until smooth.

Add in the almond milk, vanilla, honey, and chia seeds and mix until well combined.

Pour the mixture into an airtight container and refrigerate, covered for 4 hours.

Spoon the pudding into desired serving dish and top with sliced banana, roasted peanuts, and crunchy granola clusters.

Enjoy!

Berry Cheesecake Crepes

Things You Need

for 2 servings

2 cups all-purpose flour (250 g)

3 eggs

¼ cup butter (55 g), melted

3 tablespoons granulated sugar

3 cups milk (710 mL)

1 cup raspberry (125 g)

1 cup blueberry (100 g)

1 cup blackberry (150 g)

2 tablespoons lemon juice

¼ cup sugar (50 g)

¼ cup powdered sugar (40 g)

8 oz cream cheese (225 g), 1 block, softened

powdered sugar, to garnish

Instructions

In a large bowl, combine flour, eggs, butter, and sugar, stirring until ingredients are slightly mixed.

Add the milk ½ cup (120 ml) at a time, stirring vigorously, making sure the milk is completely incorporated into the batter and that the batter is smooth before adding more milk.

Repeat with the rest of the milk. The batter should be very liquidy and have no lumps.

In a pan over medium heat, pour ⅓ cup (95 g) of the batter in the center and swirl the batter around the edges of the pan until set.

To know when the crepe is ready to flip, lift up one of the edges about ⅓ of the way. The bottom side should be golden brown. Flip the crepe.

Cook until the edges are starting to slightly crisp.

Remove from heat and cover with a paper towel to make sure the crepes stay moist.

In a pot over medium heat, combine all the berries with the lemon juice and the sugar, stirring until the mixture comes to a boil.

Cook for about 2 minutes, then remove from heat and cool completely.

Mix the cream cheese with the powdered sugar until smooth.

Spread half of the cream cheese mixture on one side of the crepe.

Spread half of the berries on top of the cream cheese.

Fold the crepe over the berries, then fold in half.

Repeat with the other crepe.

Serve with powdered sugar.

Enjoy!

Banana Berry Fruit Salad

Things You Need

for 4 servings

3 bananas, sliced

12 oz fresh strawberry (340 g), q uartered

12 oz fresh raspberry (340 g)

Dressing

3 tablespoons lime juice

1 tablespoon maple syrup

Instructions

Combine all the ingredients above in a large bowl.

Mix the dressing ingredients together and spread over fruit, mix well.

Enjoy!

Apple Pie (Macerated)

Things You Need

for 8 servings

5 lb granny smith apple (2.2 kg)

1 cup brown sugar (220 g)

¼ teaspoon fine salt

2 teaspoons ground cinnamon

⅓ cup fresh lemon juice (80 mL)

3 ½ tablespoons cornstarch, divided

3 tablespoons water

3 ½ tablespoons unsalted butter

2 premade pie crusts, rolled out into ⅛-inch (3-mm) thick

egg wash

sanding sugar, for sprinkling

Instructions

Peel and thinly slice the apples (keep the apples in a bowl of lemon water as you go to keep them from browning).

In a large bowl, toss the apples with the brown sugar, salt, cinnamon, lemon juice, and half of the cornstarch. Once the apples are well coated, let sit and macerate for 30 minutes, stirring occasionally.

Preheat the oven to 400°F (200°C).

Transfer the apples to a colander set over a medium bowl and let drain for about 15 minutes, until all of the liq uid is drawn out.

Transfer the liquid released from the apples to a small pot over low heat.

In a small bowl, mix the rest of the cornstarch and the water to make a slurry. Add the slurry to the apple liq uid and quickly stir to incorporate. Bring to a boil, then add the butter and stir until melted. Immediately remove from the heat and pour over the apples, stirring to coat.

Gently lay 1 rolled-out pie crust in a 10-inch (25-cm) pie dish.

Lay the apples in the pie crust, making sure they are flat and facing the rounded edges out in order to fit as many apples as possible in the crust. Pour any leftover liquid from the bowl over the apples.

Top with the other rolled-out pie crust. Trim the excess dough from the edges.

Press the 2 crusts together to seal, then fold the edges under. Crimp the edges.

Then brush all over with egg wash and sprinkle the with sanding sugar.

Use a paring knife to cut a few vents in the top for steam to escape.

Bake for 40-45 minutes, until golden brown.

Let cool for at least an hour

Slice and serve.

Enjoy!

Strawberry Chocolate Mousse

Things You Need

for 2 servings

6 oz dark chocolate (170 g), 72% is best

½ cup low fat milk (120 mL)

1 teaspoon pure vanilla extract

1 pinch salt

1 cup greek yogurt (285 g)

8 strawberries

Instructions

In a small saucepan, heat milk on medium-low heat until scalding around 180°F (82°C). Do not boil the milk.

Pour hot milk over chocolate.

Add vanilla and salt. Let it stand for 3 minutes to soften.

Whisk together until fully incorporated. Let cool.

Add yogurt. Whisk together until fully incorporated.

Layer chocolate in the bottom of 2 cups followed by strawberries. Repeat until the glasses are full.

Enjoy!

Fudgiest Dairy-Free Chocolate Cake

Things You Need

for 10 servings

Frosting

30 oz full-fat coconut milk (880 mL), 2 cans

3 cups dairy-free chocolate chunk (510 g)

¼ cup coconut oil (60 g), melted

2 cups powdered sugar (240 g)

Cake

3 cups whole wheat flour (390 g)

1 ½ cups dark cocoa powder (180 g)

1 cup sugar (200 g)

1 tablespoon baking soda

1 ½ teaspoons baking powder

1 pinch salt

3 cups almond milk (710 mL)

1 cup coconut oil (240 g), melted

1 ½ cups applesauce (380 g)

1 ½ cups maple syrup (505 g)

1 tablespoon apple cider vinegar

1 tablespoon vanilla extract

berry, of choice, for garnish

Instructions

In a microwave-safe measuring cup, or in a small pot on the stove, heat the coconut milk until hot, but not boiling (about 2 minutes in the microwave).

Place the dairy-free chocolate in a large bowl and pour the hot coconut milk over it, allowing the milk to melt the chocolate. Mix well to combine.

Once the chocolate is melted, add the coconut oil and powdered sugar. Beat with a hand mixer or whisk until smooth.

Cover and refrigerate overnight.

Preheat the oven to 350°F (180°C). Grease 3 separate 8-inch (20-cm) round cake pans and set aside.

In a large bowl, add the whole wheat flour, dark cocoa powder, sugar, baking soda, baking powder, and salt. Whisk to combine and set aside.

In a separate large bowl, add the almond milk, coconut oil, applesauce, maple syrup, apple cider vinegar, and vanilla extract. Whisk to combine.

In two batches, add the dry mixture to the wet mixture, folding with a spatula until combined. Some clumps are okay.

Divide the batter evenly between the 3 pre-greased cake pans and bake for 35–45 minutes, or until a toothpick comes out almost entirely clean. Cool completely.

Remove the frosting from the fridge and mix it up well.

Choose which cake will be your bottom layer and cover evenly with about 1 cup (115 G) of frosting. Top with the second layer, frosting evenly again. Add the final layer and frost the top and the sides of the cake generously, topping with berries of choice for garnish.

Enjoy!

Aunt Vivian's Sweet Potato Pie

Things You Need

for 8 servings

3 lb large sweet potato (1.3 g), 4 potatoes

1 cup unsalted butter (225 g), 2 sticks, melted

2 ½ cups sugar (500 g)

1 teaspoon ground nutmeg

1 teaspoon ground cinnamon

½ teaspoon kosher salt

4 large eggs

1 tablespoon self-rising flour

¼ cup buttermilk (60 mL)

1 teaspoon vanilla extract

1 teaspoon lemon extract

3 pies frozen prepared pie crust, unbaked

Instructions

Cook the sweet potatoes in a large pot of boiling water until fork-tender, about 25-30 minutes. Drain and let cool completely.

Preheat the oven to 365°F (185°C).

Peel the sweet potatoes, then transfer to a large bowl and mash thoroughly with an electric hand mixer or fork.

Add the melted butter, sugar, nutmeg, cinnamon, and salt. Beat to combine, then scrape down the sides of the bowl with a rubber spatula. Add the eggs, 1 at a time, beating to incorporate each addition. Add the self-rising flour, buttermilk, vanilla, and lemon extract, and beat to combine.

Divide the sweet potato filling between the frozen pie crusts and smooth the tops.

Bake for about 1 hour, until pies are set in the center. Cover the crusts with foil if it is getting too dark before the pies finish baking.

Cool the pies for 2 hours on a wire rack.

Slice and serve.

Enjoy!

Frozen Banana Ice Cream

Things You Need

for 4 servings

3 ripe bananas

1 tablespoon vanilla extract

¾ cup peanut butter (180 g)

Instructions

Peel the bananas and slice into 1-inch (2 cm) slices.

Spread the bananas on a parchment-lined baking sheet and freeze for 2 hours.

Blend the frozen banana slices in a high-speed blender until they reach a smooth consistency.

Add the vanilla and peanut butter and blend to combine.

Transfer to a bowl or container and freeze for 1 hour, or until ready to serve.

Scoop out ice cream.

Enjoy!

ANTI-COLITIS SNACKS

Almond Butter Honey Oat Bars

Things You Need

for 8 servings

2 cups rolled oats (160 g)

⅔ cup almond butter (160 g), or nut butter of choice

¼ cup honey (85 g), or maple syrup

Instructions

In a medium bowl, add oats, nut butter, and honey or maple syrup, and mix until well combined.

Spray baking dish with cooking spray. Pour in mixture and spread evenly.

Cover and place in freezer until firm.

Cut into bars. Keep in the fridge until ready to eat.

Enjoy!

Baked Cinnamon Apple Chips

Things You Need

for 1 serving

1 golden delicious apple, thinly sliced

¼ teaspoon ground cinnamon

1 pinch salt

Instructions

Preheat oven to 250°F (120°C).

Place apple slices on a parchment paper-lined baking sheet and sprinkle with cinnamon and salt.

Bake for 40 minutes, until the apples are slightly browned.

Cool completely before serving.

Enjoy!

Sweet Potato Wedges

Things You Need

for 3 servings

3 medium sweet potatoes

⅓ cup olive oil (80 mL)

1 teaspoon salt

½ teaspoon pepper

2 tablespoons fresh rosemary, finely chopped

Instructions

Preheat oven to 400°F (200°C).

Thoroughly wash sweet potatoes. Slice in half, then into wedges.

Toss wedges in olive oil and seasonings.

Place on a baking sheet, skin side down.

Bake 30-40 minutes.

Enjoy!

Garlic Parmesan Roasted Chickpeas

Things You Need

for 4 servings

15 oz chickpeas (400 g), 1 can, drained and rinsed

1 tablespoon olive oil

2 cloves garlic, minced

1 teaspoon italian herb

2 tablespoons grated parmesan cheese

Instructions

Preheat oven to 400°F (200°C).

Carefully dry the chickpeas. Removing the skins is optional and they will come off easily. The drier you get them, the crunchier they'll be!

In a medium bowl, add dried chickpeas, olive oil, garlic powder, herbs and parmesan. Toss well to coat evenly.

Spread chickpeas out on a parchment paper-lined baking sheet.

Roast for 15-20 minutes.

Mix around on baking sheet and roast for additional 15-20 minutes, or until golden.

Cool for 5-10 minutes.

Enjoy!

Classic Hummus

Things You Need

for 2 cups

14 oz chickpeas (395 g), 1 can

2 cloves garlic

¼ cup tahini sauce (60 g)

2 tablespoons lemon juice

1 teaspoon cumin

½ teaspoon red pepper flakes

½ teaspoon salt

½ teaspoon black pepper

2 tablespoons extra virgin olive oil

2 tablespoons water

fresh parsley, chopped, to serve

Instructions

Add chickpeas, garlic, tahini, lemon juice, and seasonings to the bowl of a 2-q uart food processor. Blend until smooth.

While blending, slowly add in the olive oil and water until hummus is creamy and smooth.

Garnish with additional red pepper flakes, chopped parsley, and a drizzle of olive oil.

Enjoy!

Spicy Roasted Chickpeas

Things You Need

for 1 serving

15 oz chickpeas (425 g), 1 can, drained and rinsed

1 tablespoon olive oil

1 teaspoon ground cumin

1 teaspoon chili powder

½ teaspoon cayenne pepper

½ teaspoon salt

Instructions

Preheat oven to 400°F (200°C).

Carefully dry the chickpeas. Removing the skins is optional and they will come off easily. The drier you get them, the crunchier they'll be!

In a medium bowl, add dried chickpeas, olive oil, cumin, chili powder, cayenne pepper and salt. Toss well to coat evenly.

Spread chickpeas out on a parchment paper-lined baking sheet.

Roast for 15-20 minutes.

Mix around on baking sheet and roast for additional 15-20 minutes, or until browned.

Cool for 5-10 minutes.

Enjoy!

Make-Ahead Mixed Berry Parfaits

Things You Need

for 1 serving

½ cup yogurt (125 g)

½ cup granola (60 g)

1 cup mixed berries (100 g)

honey, optional

Instructions

In a jar, layer yogurt, granola, and berries. Top with honey (optional).

Refrigerate up to 2 days. If you don't want soggy granola, wait til you're ready to eat the parfait to add it.

Enjoy!

Black Bean & Quinoa Snack Bowl

Things You Need

for 1 serving

¼ cup quinoa (40 g), cooked

¼ cup black beans (40 g)

¼ cup red onion (35 g), diced

2 tablespoons corn

1 tablespoon fresh cilantro

1 teaspoon lime juice

salt, to taste

pepper, to taste

Instructions

Combine all ingredients in a small bowl.

Mix until combined and serve.

Enjoy!

Baked Chicken Fries

Things You Need

for 4 servings

4 boneless, skinless chicken breasts

2 cups plain breadcrumbs (230 g)

1 cup flour (125 g)

5 eggs, beaten

1 teaspoon salt

½ teaspoon garlic powder

½ teaspoon onion powder

½ teaspoon paprika

½ teaspoon dried basil

½ teaspoon dried oregano

½ teaspoon pepper

Instructions

Preheat oven to 375°F (190°C).

Slice chicken breast in half, and cut into thin strips about the thickness of a french fry.

Season bread crumbs with salt, garlic powder, onion powder, paprika, dried basil, dried oregano, and pepper. Mix well.

Dredge chicken strips in the flour first, then cover in egg, and coat with bread crumbs.

Place on a baking sheet lined with parchment paper and bake for 20 minutes, flipping halfway.

Enjoy!

Banana Berry Fruit Salad

Things You Need

for 4 servings

3 bananas, sliced

12 oz fresh strawberry (340 g), quartered

12 oz fresh raspberry (340 g)

Dressing

3 tablespoons lime juice

1 tablespoon maple syrup

Instructions

Combine all the Things You Need above in a large bowl.

Mix the dressing Things You Need together and spread over fruit, mix well.

Enjoy!

Keto-Friendly Flatbread

Things You Need

for 1 flatbread

1 cup shredded mozzarella cheese (100 g)

1 tablespoon cream cheese

1 large egg, beaten

¼ cup almond flour (30 g)

2 cloves garlic, minced

½ teaspoon dried oregano

½ teaspoon dried thyme

1 teaspoon fresh rosemary, minced

salt, to taste

pepper, to taste

Instructions

In a medium bowl, combine the mozzarella and cream cheese. Microwave in 30-second intervals, stirring in between, until the cheese is fully melted and the consistency is smooth, about 1 minute total.

Let the mixture cool for a few minutes to prevent the egg from scrambling, then add the egg, almond flour, garlic, oregano, thyme, rosemary, salt, and pepper, and stir until thoroughly combined.

Preheat the oven to 350°F (180°C). Line a baking sheet with parchment paper or grease with nonstick spray.c

Transfer the mixture to the baking sheet. Press and flatten firmly into an even layer about ¼-½-inch (½-1 ¼ cm) thick.

Bake for 10-15 minutes, until golden brown.

Serve as desired: slice into chips, cut into breadsticks, or top with your favorite sauce and toppings to make a pizza.

Enjoy!

Raspberry Sorbet

Things You Need

for 2 servings

1 lb frozen raspberry (455 g)

¼ cup honey (85 g), or preferred sweetener

Instructions

Blend all ingredients in a food processor or high-speed blender until thoroughly combined.

Pour into a rectangular loaf pan and smooth into an even layer.

Freeze for 2 hours, or until frozen but still a little soft for scooping. (If freezing overnight, cover with a lid or plastic wrap, but let it sit out at room temperature for about 5-10 minutes before scooping.)

Scoop into a bowl.

Enjoy!

After School Banana Roll-Ups

Things You Need

for 1 serving

1 flour tortilla, burrito sized

2 tablespoons almond butter

1 banana, peeled

Instructions

Evenly spread almond butter over one side of the tortilla.

Place banana along one edge of the tortilla, and roll up.

Slice the roll into small pieces.

Enjoy!

6-Minute Apple Crisp

Things You Need

for 1 serving

Apple Pie Filling

1 honeycrisp apple

1 tablespoon water

¼ teaspoon cinnamon

1 tablespoon brown sugar

1 teaspoon all purpose flour

1 pinch kosher salt

Crumble Topping

3 tablespoons old fashion oat

1 tablespoon all purpose flour

1 tablespoon brown sugar

¼ teaspoon cinnamon, plus more for topping

1 pinch kosher salt

2 tablespoons unsalted butter, softened

whipped cream, for serving

Instructions

Make the filling: Peel the apple, then dice into small pieces, avoiding the core.

Add the apple and water to a large, microwave-safe mug. Microwave for 1 minute, until the apple is tender.

Remove from the microwave and stir in the cinnamon, brown sugar, flour, and salt.

Make the crumble topping: In a small bowl, mix together the oats, flour, brown sugar, cinnamon, and salt with a fork. Mash in the butter until crumbly chunks form.

Spoon the topping over the apple mixture. Microwave on high power for 3–4 minutes, until the filling is juicy and bubbling and the topping is golden brown.

Top with whipped cream and a sprinkle of cinnamon, then serve.

Enjoy!

Asparagus Fries

Things You Need

for 1 serving

1 bundle asparagus

1 cup almond (140 g), chopped

⅓ cup parmesan cheese (35 g)

1 tablespoon garlic powder

2 tablespoons dried oregano

1 teaspoon salt

1 teaspoon pepper

2 eggs

Greek Yogurt Chive Dip

1 cup plain greek yogurt (285 g)

1 tablespoon lemon juice

2 tablespoons chives

¼ teaspoon salt

¼ teaspoon pepper

Instructions

Preheat oven to 425°F (220°C).

Cut off about 1-2 inches (2.5-5 cm) of asparagus ends. Set aside.

In a large bowl combine crushed almonds, parmesan, garlic powder, oregano, salt, and pepper.

Whisk eggs in a shallow bowl or dish.

Dip asparagus in eggs, coating evenly, and then toss with the crushed almond mixture.

Place on a baking sheet lined with parchment paper in a single layer. Bake for 15-20 minutes, flipping halfway.

Prepare dip while fries are baking. Combine all dip Things You Need in a small bowl and set aside in the refrigerator until ready to use.

Enjoy!

SECTION 5: FINALLY

Colitis, an increasingly prevalent disorder, manifests when the mucosal lining of the colon becomes inflamed, either suddenly or persistently. Symptoms include watery diarrhea, gut discomfort, tenesmus, urgency, fever, subjective weariness, or blood in the stool. Various factors can trigger colitis, such as infection, autoimmune conditions, ischemia, toxin exposure, immunodeficiency, and radiation exposure.

This condition presents a complex challenge, requiring a multifaceted approach to diagnosis and treatment. Novel techniques and therapies have emerged to address colitis, reflecting ongoing efforts to improve patient outcomes. Understanding the fundamental and clinical aspects of colitis is crucial for achieving successful management.

In this endeavor, we explore the diagnosis and treatment of colitis, highlighting the indispensable role of the interprofessional healthcare team in caring for affected individuals. By providing a comprehensive overview of colitis, encompassing its etiology, epidemiology, pathophysiology, assessment, treatment modalities, and potential complications, we aim to empower healthcare professionals to enhance patient care and outcomes.

The Author's Suggestion

As chronic colitis becomes increasingly common in Western countries, it presents a complex puzzle for both medical professionals and individuals affected by the condition. Despite extensive research, the precise triggers and mechanisms underlying this chronic inflammation of the colon remain elusive. However, healthcare experts suggest that the modern Western diet may play a significant role in its development.

The typical Western dietary pattern, characterized by the consumption of inflammatory processed foods and high levels of saturated fats, is believed to contribute to ongoing, low-grade inflammation within the digestive tract. This chronic inflammation, in turn, can exacerbate symptoms and worsen the progression of colitis.

In light of this, adopting an anti-inflammatory approach to nutrition may offer a promising strategy for managing chronic colitis and supporting intestinal health. Incorporating whole foods that are rich in anti-inflammatory compounds, such as fruits, vegetables, whole grains, and fatty fish, can help reduce inflammation and promote healing within the gut.

Additionally, emphasizing the consumption of unsaturated fats, found in sources like olive oil, nuts, and avocados, over saturated fats from processed and fried foods, may further mitigate inflammation and support overall digestive wellness.

While dietary modifications alone may not be sufficient to entirely prevent or cure chronic colitis, they can serve as an important component of a comprehensive treatment plan. By making mindful choices about the foods we eat, we can empower ourselves to take an active role in managing our health and promoting the well-being of our intestines.